THE

AIDS

PLAGUE

By Dr. James McKeever, Ph.D.

Omega Publications
P. O. Box 4130
Medford, OR 97501

THE AIDS EPIDEMIC

Copyright © 1986 by James M. McKeever

Printed in the United States of America
First printing December, 1985

Omega Publications
P. O. Box 4130
Medford, Oregon 97501 (U.S.A.)

ISBN 0-86694-104-5 (Softback)
ISBN 0-86694-105-3 (Hardback)

TABLE OF CONTENTS

FOREWORD

Over the centuries, plagues of one type or another, with their suffering and death, have come and gone. Some have been produced by bacteria, such as bubonic plague (the Black Plague). Others have a virus origin (small pox). Certain of the plagues have been man-made, such as the "Battle of London" or Hiroshima.

How man has recognized, diagnosed, reacted to and finally overcome these enormous disasters has been a subject for people like you and me, as well as historians, to consider, study and marvel at.

There is nothing to suggest that hiding the facts concerning a plague, delay in giving information or outright lying has in any way lessened the seriousness or the consequences. Actually, such tactics may have worsened the results of a plague.

The author has faced what appears to be the newest plague--AIDS, which has come on the world scene in the early '80s--with honesty, candor and realism. It is little wonder that, with such an approach, some of the facts are shocking, to say the least.

However, since preventive measures may be helpful, the presentation of the facts is certainly justified. The writer has done a remarkable job, in taking the very technical information concerning the immune mechanism and the etiologic virus causing AIDS, and translating them into terms that are understandable to the lay person.

How we fight off disease--the immune system--is enormously complex. The virus appears to heavily damage this system, resulting in the symptom complex we call AIDS. The author's problems are compounded by the fact that scientists in the field are at present unsure of many of the bits of information. This uncertainty is reflected in their communications and answers to questions. This frequently gives the impression that they are hiding or suppressing information.

As country after country reports cases, it is apparent that AIDS is a worldwide plague. The full gravity of the situation is just now beginning to be understood. The writer looks at possible benefits that might occur in morality, as well as the impact on the world economy. He examines the possibility that AIDS will drive people to the God of the Bible. In a sense, he echoes what Joshua said so many centuries ago, "Choose you this day whom you will serve, but as for me and my house, we will serve the Lord."

In the final analysis, I believe the only adequate solution for AIDS is a vital faith in the resurrected Christ!

Ralph L. Byron, M.D., F.A.C.S.

Former Chief of Surgery, City of Hope Hospital
Diplomate of the American Board of Surgery

November, 1985

INTRODUCTION

I have always disliked long introductions in books, so I will try to make this as brief as possible.

Introductions are supposed to tell you why the author wrote the book. In this case, that should be fairly obvious. I believe the AIDS epidemic will spread to major plague proportions, since already 1 to 3 million Americans have it and are infecting others, in most cases without even knowing it. The number of those infected is doubling every year, and so this epidemic could endanger a significant portion of the population of the U.S.

AIDS is not a homosexual disease. Based on the information available to date, in the end far more heterosexuals will die from it than homosexuals. I felt a need to tell people how they could protect themselves and their families from acquiring the dreaded disease of AIDS.

I sincerely hope that the information in this book will cause our governmental agencies to begin to treat this as a major health hazard to our nation and to take appropriate emergency actions.

If I have helped you as an individual or our nation as a whole, the efforts and energy of producing this work will have been worth it.

New research information on AIDS is coming forth daily, and so no book is adequate to keep you current on this critical subject. Therefore, to present the findings as they occur, I have teamed up with René Baxter, a brilliant researcher, to produce a monthly newsletter called THE AIDS UPDATE. This will be an on-going supplement to this book.

I would encourage you to read the book carefully, because it could save your life or the lives of your loved ones.

Sincerely yours,

Dr. James McKeever, Ph. D.

ACKNOWLEDGEMENTS

In researching this book, I have had personal interviews with a number of the leading researchers and thinkers concerning AIDS and have received input from many others. I could never acknowledge everyone who has helped me in this work, but I would specifically like to thank:

Dr. Margaret Bottiger, Sweden
  National Bacteriological Laboratory
Dr. Ralph Byron, City of Hope
  Chief of Surgery
Dr. James Curran
  Centers for Disease Control
Dr. Dean Echenverg
  San Francisco Health Department
Dr. Robert Gallo
  National Cancer Institute
Dr. Michael Gottlieb
  UCLA Immunologist
Dr. John Grauerholz, EIR
  Pathologist and AIDS Expert
Dr. Phil Markham
  Litton Research
Dr. Lue Montagnier, Paris
  Pasteur Institute
Dr. Richard O'Toole
  Internist and Virus Expert
Dr. Robert Redfield
  Walter Reed Army Medical Center
Dr. Bijan Safai
  Sloan-Kettering Cancer Center

Dr. John Seale, London
Venereal Disease Expert
Dr. Paul Volberding, San Francisco
Head of the AIDS Clinic

Of course, these outstanding men and women do not agree with every word in this book. They do not even agree completely with each other. But each of them have made a valuable contribution to this book.

I am especially indebted to René Baxter, who has been superb in his role as research assistant. He has become one of the most knowledgeable men concerning AIDS in this capacity and has done an outstanding job. I also appreciate the excellent work in typing, editing and typesetting the book done by Jim Andrews and Annette Wright.

Most of all, my appreciation goes to my wonderful wife, Jeani. She was the prime editor of the book and provided me suggestions and insights. At the same time, she gave me encouragement and inspiration. She has been the perfect wife and co-laborer.

I also want to thank all of those unseen thousands who will read this book and recommend it to others. They (you) will play a valuable role in spreading the word and helping to stop the spread of the AIDS plague.

James McKeever
P.O. Box 1788
Medford, OR 97501

1
PLAGUE, EPIDEMICS AND PANDEMICS

There have been many epidemics (or plagues) that have changed the course of history. These have brought death and misery to humankind throughout the centuries. Most people today think that these plagues are a thing of the dim past and something that could not happen now.

However, there is a plague that is just in its inception that we believe will prove to be a history-changing one, and that is the plague of AIDS.

It is our best forecast that, within twelve years, 20 to 25 percent of the population of the United States will die or be dying of AIDS. That may be somewhat startling at first, but in the next two chapters we will give hard evidence to back up that conclusion. We are not trying to be sensational; we are trying to be realistic. We believe that the facts will support this, as you will see in ensuing chapters.

THE SPANISH FLU PLAGUE

Plagues have occurred in this century. Most people today are not aware of the fact that in the United States in 1918 and 1919,

U.S. POPULATION IN 1920 – 92 MILLION+

there was an epidemic of the Spanish flu (influenza) that killed 500,000 people. Ultimately, worldwide, it caused the death of 20 million people. It was not until 1933 that an influenza virus was identified as the cause of that disease.

According to W.I.B. Beveridge, author of INFLUENZA: THE LAST GREAT PLAGUE: in Samoa, 25 percent of the people died; the Eskimos in Alaska suffered terribly from the Spanish flu, and some entire villages were wiped out totally, while others lost their entire adult population.[1] He points out that in Nome, Alaska, 176 out of 300 Eskimos died (59 percent). He informs us that the disease caused havoc in India when an estimated 5 million people died. In Punjab, the streets were littered with the dead, and at railroad stations the trains had to be cleared of dead and dying passengers before they could continue down the track. The burial grounds there were covered with corpses. All of this happened just a little more than sixty years ago.

This was a "pandemic," which is a plague (epidemic) of worldwide proportions. This pandemic did not care about social or economic classes: everyone from kings to beggars suffered. And remember, this great visitation of death happened less than seventy years ago, in this century. Pandemics are not events of the remote past; they can occur even today.

William Beveridge points out that in 1957 a pandemic of the Asian flu began in

China. In the United States, the attack rate of people contracting the disease the following winter was from 50 to 70 percent of the people from ten to twenty years old, and 20 to 40 percent of the people from twenty to fifty years old. Although the disease mortality was only 60,000 deaths, the number affected by it was significantly higher. If it had been 100-percent fatal, 30 to 60 percent of the U.S. population would have died from it.

In 1968, there appeared the Hong Kong flu, which came to the United States in the following winter (1969), and all age groups were attacked. The mortality in the United States was estimated to be around 80,000 people, with 30 to 40 percent of the people becoming infected. What would have occurred if it had been 100-percent fatal?

In times past, there have been numerous other major pandemics of flu. These occurred in:

1889	1857	1847
1830	1802	1781

All of these crises have occurred within the last two hundred years. These pandemics were caused by a virus which was spread from person to person via the respiratory route only.

We forecast that AIDS will be a pandemic, also spread by a virus from person to person in various ways.

THE BUBONIC PLAGUE

This is also called the black death plague, probably because of the dark areas of skin on the dying victims. The black death plague was one of the most terrible plagues in the history of Europe, killing an estimated 25 million persons.

In this plague, the disease was initially spread to man by means of infected rats or rat fleas. Subsequent spread was from man to man by way of infected pulmonary secretions. It was characterized by fever, swelling of the lymph nodes throughout the body, and pneumonia.

Traders brought the disease to Europe in the early 1300's. It had struck in Sicily in 1347, and spread across the Mediterranean to strike England and France in 1348. It is estimated that 30 percent to possibly 50 percent of the English people died of the plague. In Bristol, the living were hardly able to bury the dead. In three years, the black plague may have killed at least 30-40 percent of the population of Europe.

After 1400, the black plague returned many times to plague Europe, until about 1700. The black death hastened the breakup of medieval society. Agriculture came to a near standstill. The production of goods fell. Goods became scarce and, thus, prices rose (inflation).

Because laborers were scarce, wages rose. This caused revolts to break out in England, France and elsewhere. This pandemic (plague) led to hysteria.

Today the bubonic plague is rare and can be treated with antibiotics. However, at one time it was a history-changing plague.

PLAGUES IN EGYPT

In the Old Testament of the Bible, there is recorded a succession of calamities (plagues) that God inflicted on the Egyptians to win freedom for the Israelite slaves. Each time when Moses asked the Pharaoh to let God's people go, the monarch merely increased their toil. The ten plagues that occurred were as follows:

1. The water of the Nile turned to blood.

2. Frogs infested the land.

3. Lice (or gnats) appeared throughout the land.

4. Great swarms of insects came.

5. The livestock of the Egyptians died.

6. Boils broke out on man and beast.

7. There was hail mixed with fire.

8. Locusts darkened the land.

9. There were three days of darkness.

10. The firstborn of the Egyptians (and disobedient Israelites) died.

After the death of the firstborn, the Pharaoh told Moses that the Israelites could leave.

These plagues also were of a history-changing nature. If the Israelite slaves had remained there in Egypt for the next two to three thousand years, history would have been quite different indeed. Vast percentages of the population did not die during these plagues in Egypt, but it was still history-changing in scope.

AIDS: A GROWING PANDEMIC

It has been recognized that AIDS is an epidemic, and I believe it will be a history-changing pandemic or plague. On a worldwide basis, it is as much a hetero-sexual disease as it is homosexual, so heterosexuals should not sit back smug and unconcerned. When the AIDS epidemic began in the U.S., a very small percentage of the cases involved heterosexuals. By the end of 1985, this had grown to the point at which almost 40 percent of the new cases were heterosexual.[2] Very soon, the vast majority of the new cases in the U.S. will be heterosexual, as is the situation in Africa, where AIDS began.

The April 29, 1985, edition of NEWSWEEK, quoted Dr. Bijan of New York's Memorial Sloan-Kettering Cancer Center as saying:[3]

"The data you hear on heterosexual infection is exactly what we were hearing in '81 on homosexuals. You have a very few heterosexuals coming down with the disease, but in the coming years, those numbers will grow. It's already happening."

This deadly AIDS virus is spreading across the world. The following table shows the number of cases reported in various countries:

Table 1.1

Country	End of 1984 Cases Reported	6/30/85 Cases Reported
France	260	392
Brazil	182	
Canada	165	
West Germany	135	220
United Kingdom	108	176
Belgium	65	99
Netherlands	42	66
Switzerland	41	63
Denmark	34	48
Spain	18	38
Sweden	16	27
Italy	14	52
Austria	13	18
Mexico	12	
Argentina	11	
Japan	3	
Asia	1	

According to Dr. Margaret Bottiger of Sweden's National Bacteriological Laboratory, Europe is about two and a half years behind the United States in the number of AIDS cases, but it is rapidly catching up.

There is no need to panic over AIDS. Panic is an emotional state which either immobilizes or leads to irrational action. However, there is a need for grave concern. Intense concern will motivate us to meaningful action.

Up until now the media and the government have almost tried to "cover up" AIDS for fear that the public will panic. In the meantime, at least 1 million Americans have been infected with AIDS, and each of them could be infecting others. This number is an estimate by Dr. James Curran, who heads the Task Force on AIDS for the respected Centers For Disease Control (CDC). He bases this estimate on the number of units of blood in blood banks which contained the antibody to the AIDS virus. These are Americans who have the AIDS virus, but the symptoms have not yet appeared. When the symptoms do appear, and these people are terminally ill, then and only then will the CDC classify them as AIDS "cases." In my humble opinion, with a million or more infected, this already should be classified as a national health emergency.

A military base goes into "Condition Yellow" when the enemy is in the vicinity. They then go to "Condition Orange" when the enemy comes closer. They finally go to

"Condition Red" when harm is imminent. There is no panic at a Red Alert, but there is serious concern and acute alertness.

It is time to declare a state of national health emergency concerning AIDS. There is no need to panic, but there is a need to alert people and to have some concentrated action.

The AIDS epidemic is in its infancy at this point in the United States (at the end of 1985). In Chapter 3, we will examine the facts on which we base our conclusion that this will become a pandemic of major proportions. However, we need to first look at the facts about AIDS and the AIDS virus, so that we will be able to base our conclusions on concrete information rather than rumor and hearsay.

2
FACTS ABOUT AIDS

There are many stories, news releases and rumors floating around concerning AIDS. Some of these are true and some are false. We need to be able to separate fact from fiction and to ascertain what the real facts are concerning AIDS.

There is very little literature on AIDS from which we can discern the facts. What is in a written form at present comes from periodicals. Thus, for us to research the true facts concerning AIDS has involved a great deal of time and interviews. We have interviewed researchers in the Walter Reed Hospital, the Centers for Disease Control, the National Cancer Institute, Litton Research Institute and many others.

Frequently, we would talk to one researcher who could answer some questions and then he would give us the name of someone else who could handle the questions that he was unable to answer. I am in debt to these outstanding men for their wisdom and knowledge. They were able to help us separate fantasy from fact.

First we will start with the name "AIDS" itself. This stands for Acquired Immune Deficiency Syndrome. "Acquired" means that it is something that one gets. The disease itself is an attack on one's immune system, which makes the immune system deficient and unable to ward off even common, largely infectious, diseases.

AIDS is caused by a virus. Actually the virus' correct name is Human T-Lymphotropic Virus type III (HTLV-III). However, it is commonly called the AIDS virus. A virus can be defined as a disease-causing agent or substance that is smaller than a bacterium. A virus is a small enough disease-producing agent that it will pass through a porous porcelain filter that would hold back bacteria and other larger microorganisms. Viruses cannot be seen under conventional microscopes but can be observed with electron microscopes.

The AIDS virus attacks the body's immune system. Our immune system protects us from foreign agents capable of producing disease or illness within our body. The immune system is able to recognize these foreign substances and then organize itself to attack and eliminate them from the body.

Our immune system is not a single organ, but involves many parts of the body. For example, the skin protects us from the invasion of all sorts of bacteria, chemicals, and microorganisms that exist within our environment. The liver, bone marrow, lymph system, lungs, thymus gland and spleen all play very essential roles in our immune system. It is this system that produces the white blood cells which circulate through our body and attack foreign substances. The AIDS virus attacks the lymph system, primarily certain lymphocytes.

The name AIDS (Acquired Immune Deficiency Syndrome) is imperfect, because it implies that the virus only attacks the immune system. That is not true. Although it primarily attacks the immune system, it can directly attack the brain or the respiratory system. Dr. John Seale reports this in the EXECUTIVE INTELLIGENCE REVIEW (EIR):[1]

"Look, it's not only a question of immune deficiency, but it attacks the brain directly! We have done post-mortems, where the brain has been shot. This is what is referred to as dementia. Bob Gallo has done work on this. There's the San Francisco group, of Jay Levy, a virologist there, at San Francisco General Hospital. Both of these have published papers, I know their work, about how the virus hits the brain as well. So, in the first report, you get people who are dying of brain disease, without AIDS, as AIDS is defined by the CDC! The problem is, it picks off the brain before it picks off the cells."

He also reported that the Pasteur Institute in France, in mid-September, grew AIDS virus from lungs. "This opens up a new can of worms. In later stages, it may be the case, that the virus attacks the lungs, and becomes a respiratory disease, like tuberculosis."

AIDS AND THE IMMUNE SYSTEM

In no way do we want to be too technical in this discussion, but bear with us for just a moment. The two basic lymphocytes are the "T" and "B" lymphocytes.

In a layman's summary, it works this way.   If a normal virus--of the common

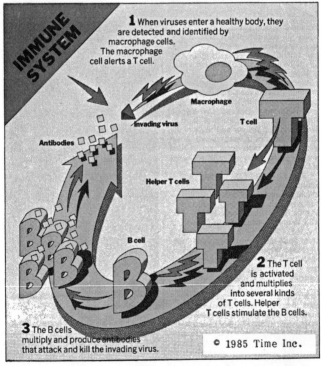

IMMUNE SYSTEM

1 When viruses enter a healthy body, they are detected and identified by macrophage cells. The macrophage cell alerts a T cell.

Macrophage

Invading virus

T cell

Antibodies

Helper T cells

B cell

2 The T cell is activated and multiplies into several kinds of T cells. Helper T cells stimulate the B cells.

3 The B cells multiply and produce antibodies that attack and kill the invading virus.

© 1985 Time Inc.

Figure 2.1

cold, for example--invades the body, these disease-fighting cells (lymphocytes) are normally activated. These are called "T" cells, helper "T" cells and "B" cells. When they recognize that a foreign substance has entered the body, they multiply and produce antibodies that will attack and kill the invading virus. This is shown in Figure 2.1.

However, the AIDS virus is treated differently by the body than any other virus. When an AIDS virus invades the body, it

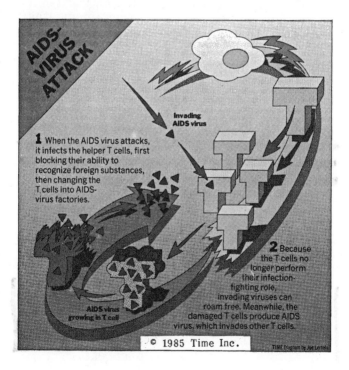

AIDS-VIRUS ATTACK

Invading AIDS virus

1 When the AIDS virus attacks, it infects the helper T cells, first blocking their ability to recognize foreign substances, then changing the T cells into AIDS-virus factories.

2 Because the T cells no longer perform their infection-fighting role, invading viruses can roam free. Meanwhile, the damaged T cells produce AIDS virus, which invades other T cells.

AIDS virus growing in T cell

© 1985 Time Inc.

TIME Diagram by Joe Lertola

Figure 2.2

goes directly to the "T" helper cells, infects them, and destroys their ability to recognize other viruses and foreign substances. The virus then actually changes the "T" cells into AIDS-virus-producing factories. Thus, these "T" cells can no longer produce "B" cells, which produce antibodies that would fight other invading viruses. They amplify AIDS rather than fighting it. This is shown in Figure 2.2.

In a very simplistic way, you could visualize it like this. Say there were a small wooden stick within your body that fought off diseases, and something came in that slowly whittled away at that stick. Ultimately, when the stick was all gone, there would be nothing left to fight invading microbes, and you would die of a disease, usually infectious and frequently exotic. We call these opportunistic diseases. In fact, no one ever dies of AIDS itself; it is simply that AIDS causes the body to be unable to fight off other viruses and bacteria.

The amount of time required to "whittle away that stick" varies with the individual, how many AIDS viruses were introduced into the body, and whether or not these viruses were introduced directly into the bloodstream.

The incubation period for AIDS ranges from two to five years. That is the amount of time from the point at which the virus is introduced into the body to the time when the AIDS symptoms begin to appear.

AIDS SYMPTOMS,
DISEASES AND MORTALITY

The symptoms of AIDS infection may be directly attributable to the HTLV-III virus, or to secondary consequences of the immune system impairment caused by infection with the AIDS virus.   The range of symptoms includes: none at all, nonspecific signs and symptoms of illness, autoimmune and neurologic disorders, a variety of oportunistic infections, and several types of malignancy.

The nonspecific syptoms include fatigue, decreased appetite, sudden weight loss, diarrhea, swollen lymph glands in the neck, armpit and groin, abdominal discomfort, dry cough, fever and other flu-like symptoms, and night sweats.   A flu-like illness frequently marks the onset of AIDS.   It is believed that one is most infectious during this period.

The single most prevalent specific symptom of AIDS is a yeast infection of the mouth and throat known as candidiasis or thrush.[2]   In full-blown AIDS, candida may cause a severe infection of the lungs.

With the immune system disabled, the AIDS sufferer is open to a variety of rare but lethal infections and malignancies.   The most common are:[3]

PNEUMOCYSTIS CARINII PNEUMONIA, "PCP", a severe virus pneumonia.   Normally, this lung infection is easily fought off by healthy people, but those with AIDS simply cannot fight off this infection.

KAPOSI'S SARCOMA, "KS", a malignant neoplasm (cancer) of the skin and internal organs.

CRYPTOCOCCOSIS, a parasitic lung infection.

TOXOPLASMOSIS, "brain rot," a parasitic, necrotic (causes tissue death) central nervous system infection which affects the brain, the eyes and the nerves.

HISTOPLASMOSIS, a parasitic lung disease that is spread through the blood system to the liver and spleen, causing enlargement, and to the adrenal glands, where it may become necrotic.

CYTOMEGALOVIRUS INFECTIONS, resulting in severe and painful enlargement in the lymph glands.

MYCOBACTERIA INFECTIONS, either atypical, tubercular, or leprositic. Associated with the AIDS outbreak has been a huge increase in the number of tuberculosis cases, especially in Africa.

HERPES INFECTIONS, severe erupting lesions of the skin, mucosa (mouth, throat, anus, etc.) and central nervous system.

In addition, two new diseases never before seen in humans have become increasingly common among AIDS sufferers:

CRYPTOSPORIDIOSIS, a severe diarrhea caused by a protozoan parasite which leads to acute malnutrition, dehydration and death. Previously found only in animals, especially calves, the first human patient was reported in 1976.   Between 1976 and 1982, seven cases of cryptosporidium infection were reported. Since 1982, the number of cases has been accelerating.[4]

ORAL VIRAL LESION (hairy leukoplakia), white, raised areas of thickening on the tongue.   Candida has been found on the surface of the lesions, and biopsies have revealed a number of virus, including papilloma, herpes and Epstein-Barr.   First identified in San Francisco in 1981, the lesion has now been reported in AIDS patients around the world.[5]

ONSET TIME: Once infected with the virus, 30 to 45 percent will become ill and be diagnosed as having AIDS within two to five years.   The majority will not show symptoms for at least five years.   The long-term prognosis for those who remain asymptomatic for five years or more is unknown due to the short period of time this disease has been under observation.[6]

MORTALITY: Once the symptoms appear and a diagnosis of AIDS is made, 60 percent die within the first year, 75 percent die within the first two years, 85 percent die within the first three years, and 100 percent die within five years after initial diagnosis.[7]

THE AIDS DIAGNOSTICS

When the AIDS virus enters the body, a special antibody is produced to try to fight

the AIDS virus. Unfortunately, this antibody
does not kill the AIDS virus, but the antibody remains in the lymphocytes of the
infected individual. A blood test has been
developed to test for this antibody. The
technical name for this blood test is a test
for the HTLV-III antibody. Many call it the
AIDS Antibody test. In this work, we will
shorten it to the "AA (AIDS Antibody) blood
test." This will tell a medical professional
whether a human has had the AIDS virus
enter and infect his body.

This blood test will progressively become
more popular, in my opinion, and individuals
who potentially could be exposed to AIDS,
or give AIDS to others, may begin to be
tested frequently. Already those entering
the armed services, as well as all existing
service personnel, are being tested for
AIDS. Why are they doing this? Perhaps
the federal government knows something that
it is not passing along to the public!

Eventually, food handlers, child care
workers, blood bank employes and others in
critical occupations may also be required to
take this blood test. However, we need to
realize that even this blood test is not 100
percent certain; it will catch only approximately 95 percent of those infected with
AIDS, under rigid laboratory conditions, and
probably less under blood bank conditions.

From an official document of the
Department of Human Resources--Oregon
State Health Division, we read the
following:[8]

The acquired immune deficiency syndrome (AIDS) is a serious illness resulting from failure of an important part of the patient's immune system. This failure is thought to be caused by infection with a newly recognized virus, the Human T-Lymphotrophic Virus III, also known as HTLV-III. . . .

THERE IS, AT PRESENT, NO DIAGNOSTIC LABORATORY TEST FOR AIDS. In other words, the determination of whether or not a person has AIDS depends upon thorough medical evaluation and tests for the infections or cancer that occur in AIDS patients. . . .

The HTLV-III antibody test is a test for antibody produced by an exposed person's immune system against the virus that is thought to cause AIDS. It is not a test for the virus itself.

The official document goes on to give warnings about the HTLV-III antibody test (the AIDS Antibody--AA blood test) and really discourages individuals from taking the test. It says:

If the fact that you have had an HTLV-III antibody test becomes part of your medical record, it could influence your health or life insurance company and adversely affect your insurability.

Rather than discouraging people from being tested for AIDS, I think that government agencies should encourage the test.

However, as we said, this test is not 100 percent reliable, especially since it does not test for the AIDS virus directly. Because this test is not perfect, it will not separate out all of the blood in a blood bank that has the AIDS virus in it.   Therefore, for hemophiliacs, the hospitals bring plasma to be given to them to 60°C (140°F) and hold it there for several hours.   Then and only then are they sure that any AIDS viruses have been killed. Formerly, they took the blood to 56°C (133°F) and held it there for ten minutes, but they have found that they must take the blood to a higher temperature and hold it there longer.

However, this is only done for hemophiliacs, not for regular patients who need blood transfusions.   The reason that blood banks do not "pasteurize" the plasma for all patients is that this pasteurization process destroys the red blood cells.   Hemophiliacs do not need the red blood cells, whereas regular patients do.

THE TWO STAGES OF AIDS

We can and, in fact, must divide the AIDS disease into two distinct stages:

AIDS--STAGE 1:   This is the period from the time a person is infected with the AIDS virus until the symptoms actually occur.   Some medical authorities call this pre-AIDS or AIDS Related Complex (ARC). However, this is simply sugarcoating the problem. These people have been infected with AIDS and can infect others.

AIDS--STAGE 2:   This is the terminal stage of AIDS, which covers the period from the time when the symptoms appear until the patient dies. This is usually two to four years. It is the AIDS--STAGE 2 patients who are classified as "AIDS cases" in most of the literature. No one has a method of counting all the AIDS--STAGE 1 cases.

Infected with AIDS	AIDS Symptoms Appear	Death because of AIDS
AIDS--STAGE 1 (incubation period) can infect others	AIDS--STAGE 2 (AIDS cases)	

Figure 2.3

There are a minimum of 1 million people in America today in AIDS--STAGE 1. This is based on the blood banks testing all of their blood with the AIDS Antibody (AA) test.

Some scientists feel that not all of these people with AIDS--STAGE 1 will develop the symptoms.   Some of them guess as low as 5-20 percent will develop symptoms. Other scientists feel that, given enough time, **all** of the people with AIDS--STAGE 1 will ultimately come down with the symptoms and move into AIDS--STAGE 2.   I would agree with the second group.

In actual fact, there is not enough data for anyone to claim that only a small percentage of the people with AIDS--STAGE 1 will move into AIDS--STAGE 2.   To prove this, they would have to have, say one hundred people who tested positive on the HTLV-III blood test and follow them for ten years.   AIDS has not been around that long, so the guesses of 5-20 percent are truly "hopes" and "guesses" and are not based on facts.

One factual clue we have is the VISNA virus in sheep.   It is essentially AIDS in sheep.   It, too, is a slow virus.   Every infected sheep dies in two-thirds the lifetime of an uninfected sheep.   With sheep, it is spread by respiratory transmission.   Even though scientists do not agree (yet), the facts that we have would lead us to conclude that all of the people in STAGE 1 will eventually move into AIDS--STAGE 2.

What scientists do agree on is that those with AIDS--STAGE 1 can infect other people.   Those who test positive on the AIDS Antibody blood test, according to the best information at this point in time, do have the AIDS virus in their bodies and they have AIDS--STAGE 1.

HOW IS AIDS TRANSMITTED?

There is much confusion over the subject of how AIDS is transmitted, but the summary of the research that has been done to date indicates that:

AIDS IS SPREAD BY THE TRANSFER OF BODY FLUIDS.

According to our knowledge at present, the way AIDS is spread is by the transference of body fluids. It is not spread by a handshake, by objects handled by people with AIDS, or by a kiss on the cheek. This would be considered "casual contact." However, there are many ways that body fluids can be transferred that some may unfortunately consider "casual." Passionate kissing is not casual contact, because body fluids are transferred.

To date, the primary way that AIDS is spread is through a sex act. This can be either by homosexual or heterosexual activity. AIDS is not a homosexual disease. Many homosexuals have acquired AIDS because of its initial introduction into the homosexual community. Because of its long incubation period, one individual could infect hundreds of gays while he was in AIDS-- STAGE 1, before he even knew he had the disease. One of the reasons it spread so rapidly through the gay community is because it tends to be a very promiscuous community.

In what population center would you think the highest percentage of the people have AIDS? San Francisco or New York? Neither of these; rather, it is Belle Glade, Florida, an isolated, rural town of 17,000 population, located in the center of the state. In the last three years, almost 40 cases have been documented. Health officials are investigating Belle Glade in an effort to discover why this apparently heterosexual town has been hit so hard.

In Africa, where AIDS began and is in epidemic proportions, it is almost universally a heterosexual disease. In the central African countries of Zaire, Rwanda, and Burundi, it affects women and men in approximately equal numbers. According to a Canadian researcher working in East Africa, "Prostitution seems to have played a key role in spreading AIDS in Africa."[9] Many of the affected males are heterosexuals who have a large number of sexual partners. Yes, indeed, women can give AIDS to men, as well as men passing it on to their female sexual partners.

AIDS is now rapidly spreading into the heterosexual community of the United States through various means. One means is by bisexual men who have contracted AIDS in the gay community, and who then knowingly or unknowingly infect prostitutes, girlfriends and their own wives with the disease.

The military high command is very concerned about AIDS being spread among the personnel of the armed forces. In Germany, it is estimated that 50-60 percent of the prostitutes have AIDS and are passing it on to servicemen who visit them.

Because of this concern, on October 15, 1985 the military began testing all recruits for AIDS. Those recruits with positive results on the AA blood test will be rejected. Then, three days later, the armed forces announced that they would test the entire 2,100,000 service men and women. Service personnel acquire AIDS in various ways, such as from prostitutes and homosexual activities. The incidence of AIDS is especially high in the Navy's submarine service.

AIDS SPREAD THROUGH BLOOD TRANSFUSIONS

Another body fluid exchange by which AIDS is transmittable is through blood transfusions, when the AIDS virus is contained within the blood that is fed intravenously into another individual. Our blood banks today have used the blood test that tests for the AIDS antibody produced when AIDS infects an individual, and they basically have discarded all of the blood that tested positive. However, there are thousands and perhaps millions of people who have had blood transfusions within the last five years. Some of them may have contracted AIDS before the blood banks began this test. Many of these thousands of people could have AIDS and could be spreading it unknowingly.

A typical example is Patrick Burk, who acquired the AIDS virus through contaminated blood. He has sexually transmitted this to his wife, Lauren, who in turn passed it on to their son, likely when he was in her womb. It was only after their son, Dwight, was diagnosed in August, 1983, (AIDS--STAGE 2) that the symptoms the parents had had (the unexplained rashes, diarrhea, and swollen lymph nodes) made sense to the doctors.

Then in December, 1984, Patrick was hospitalized with the PCP type of pneumonia which AIDS allows. On the other hand, the mother, Lauren, is in a condition that her doctors call "pre-AIDS," but that we more realistically call AIDS--STAGE 1.   This means that she has AIDS, but the full-blown AIDS symptoms have not yet appeared.

If there is any doubt that you have contracted AIDS through a blood transfusion, I would encourage you to call your doctor or your local public health officials and get a blood test so that you can be 95 percent sure, one way or the other.

AIDS TRANSMITTED BY OTHER INTRODUCTION OF BLOOD

The AIDS virus will remain "alive" for up to seven days in dried blood. This is the reason that intravenous drug users can acquire AIDS through using a common needle.

For example, if a drug user had AIDS and used a needle on Monday, some of his dried blood would remain on the needle. If, then, on Wednesday one of his friends were to use that needle, without it being totally sterilized, that friend could be introducing the AIDS virus into his or her own bloodstream. The amount of the AIDS virus, which is called the "titer," would be much smaller than in a blood transfusion. However, no matter how small the quantity of the AIDS virus that was introduced, that individual could then have AIDS--STAGE 1. It would take longer for the AIDS virus to multiply to the point at which that person would enter AIDS--STAGE 2, but the process would have started.

Many prostitutes are intravenous drug users, so this is a way that they can acquire AIDS, in addition to getting it from their male partners.

If someone had a scratch, wound, abrasion or open sore and then got blood from someone who had AIDS into that opening in his skin, the AIDS virus could come in with the blood. Here again, the quantity of the virus would be small, but nevertheless AIDS--STAGE 1 could have been entered.

AIDS TRANSMITTED BY
EXCHANGE OF OTHER BODY FLUIDS?

We have just seen that AIDS can be transmitted by an exchange of blood and by an exchange of the fluids involved in sexual relations (remember, women can give it to men). But that is not the end of the story. The AIDS virus has been found in other body fluids.

According to Dr. Dean Echenverg of the San Francisco Health Department, the AIDS virus has been found in saliva. He feels that the exchange of saliva (as occurs in deep, passionate kissing) is putting an individual at a grave risk. Washington experts agree, feeling that passionate kissing could easily transmit AIDS, since the virus is in the saliva, and they recommend that actors not allow themselves to be involved in intimate kissing scenes. This is not casual contact.

If you knew that someone had AIDS, would you want to give that individual a deep, long, "french" kiss, wherein surely you would have in your mouth some of that person's saliva, which contains the AIDS virus? The portion swallowed could potentially be killed by gastric acids, but there is frequently access to the bloodstream from the mouth via cuts, canker sores, bleeding gums or under the tongue. Since no doctor or medical authority is willing to stand up and say that AIDS cannot be transferred in this manner, it is the better part of wisdom to act as though it could be transferred this way, until it is absolutely proven otherwise.

This will probably never be proven, one way or the other. To prove it, an individual would have to have a deep kissing session with someone with AIDS and not have sex with that person. Then that individual would have to refrain from sex for at least five years, to see if the kissing and corresponding exposure to AIDS-infected saliva caused AIDS. I doubt if a volunteer for such a test will be found, and so it will remain a matter of opinion.

One thing that would help us to know whether, in fact, kissing will transfer AIDS would be for Linda Evans, who performed passionate kissing scenes with Rock Hudson, to submit to a blood test for the AIDS antibody. However, up to now she has declined to take this test.

Some researchers say things such as, "passionate kissing is not 'likely' to transmit AIDS." When pinned down about what "likely" means, they say something like "a 10 to 25 percent chance." Personally, I do not like those odds.

The quantity of the AIDS virus (the titer) is less in a unit of saliva than in the same unit of blood or semen. However, one is still bringing some quantity of the AIDS virus into his (or her) body through deep kissing an individual with AIDS and, thus, is potentially entering into AIDS--STAGE 1.

The AIDS virus has also been found in the tears of AIDS victims, according to the CDC.[10] This may not prove to be significant at all, but let us consider it briefly.

If someone with AIDS wiped a tear with his or her finger, you would not want to have that finger put in your mouth. But it would produce the same results if someone with AIDS was working in a restaurant and his eyes watered, he wiped his tears with his hands and then handled the food, say a roll which absorbed the tear, and then you ate it.   It is possible that the infection could be passed on in this manner, even though the quantity of the AIDS virus would be even less than you would take in from passionate kissing.   At this point, we just do not know how "likely" it is.   This has not yet been proven nor disproven.

We know that the AIDS virus can exist outside of the body; we just do not know how long it will live under all of the various circumstances.   In liquid blood, it will exist for many months; in dried blood, as we mentioned earlier, for a minimum of three days. The more hospitable the environment, the longer it lives.   At this point, no one knows how long it will live, say, in a piece of bread that has absorbed the tears or saliva of someone with AIDS.

Some medical authorities may scoff at the thought of acquiring AIDS through food. However,   other   medical   authorities   are equally convinced that AIDS can be spread by infected food handlers.   For example, the Abilene Medical Center in Abilene, Texas had all of its cafeteria personnel take the AA blood test.   They then laid off Johnny Warner, the only one who tested positive.

According   to   Dr.   John   Grauerholz, pathologist with EIR and outstanding AIDS expert, the Pasteur Institute in Paris performed an experiment that could shed some light on the subject. They took saliva which contained the AIDS virus and put it into a number of petri dishes. Half of the petri dishes were kept moist and half were allowed to dry. After seven days, the moist saliva had almost as many active AIDS viruses as at the beginning. The critical thing to note is that when the other samples were remoistened, after being dry for seven days, 10 percent of the AIDS viruses in them became active again. This would add validation to the concern of AIDS being transmitted through food.

AIDS IS A DREADED DISEASE

The reason we call AIDS a "dreaded disease" is that it is 100 percent fatal, and it is possible that a vaccine will never be found to cure it. On August 16, 1985, the LOS ANGELES TIMES reported this from the Associated Press Wire:[11]

> The virus suspected of causing AIDS has so many variations in its genetic structure that developing a vaccine against the disease may be difficult, if it can be done at all, researchers said Thursday.
> Scientists at the National Cancer Institute said that they looked at samples of the suspect virus found in 18 patients with AIDS or at high risk of getting the disease, and each isolated

virus showed a different variation in its genetic structure.

The study, to be published today in the journal SCIENCE, means that it could be difficult to find a common site on the viruses that could be targeted for preventive and therapeutic measures, they said.

To develop a vaccine, researchers say, they need to find a common protein region, preserved in all variations of the virus that triggers an immunologic response.

Dr. Gordon Dreesman, of the Southwest Foundation for Biomedical Research in San Antonio, Texas, was reported, by STAR magazine on September 24, 1985, as saying:[12]

"A lot of the problem in studying AIDS is that the structure of the virus seems to vary from patient to patient."

DRUGS TO HELP AIDS VICTIMS

The basic research being done today, which is occasionally reported on the nightly news, is on drugs which will slow down the body's production of the AIDS virus or help what is left of the immune system to function better. Nothing has been found which even comes close to killing the AIDS virus. There are about four or five of these drugs which have the potential to stretch out the length of AIDS--STAGE 2, but there is no hard evidence that any of them will stop it. Also, up until now, almost all of the testing has been in test tubes.

The drug HPA-23 that Rock Hudson went to France to get has now been allowed into the U.S. by the FDA on an experimental basis. It appears to reduce the "T" cell's production of the AIDS virus, but it does not stop the deterioration of the body. It also has some very bad side effects, in the liver and in elimination of blood clotting. This drug appeared to help Rock for a brief season, but in the end did not stop the terminal nature of AIDS. AIDS, like cancer and other diseases, seems to go into remission at times. Unfortunately, one of those times seems to be shortly before death.

Another of these drugs which help boost the immune system is THF, which was developed in Israel. It is a derivative from an isolated hormone from the thymus gland. It stimulates the bone marrow to produce "B" cells, helper cells. This and other such drugs assist the immune system, but the AIDS viruses are still alive and multiplying in the body.

Another drug, that was discovered in Sweden, is Trisodium Phosphoformate. Still another is Isoprinosine. These have promise to boost the body's immune system.

According to Dr. David Clausman of the Pasteur Institute in Paris, and according to a spokesman for the Centers for Disease

Control in the United States, these "immune modulators" are not the real answer for AIDS.   What is needed is something that kills the AIDS virus.   They asserted that if you want to treat the patient, you have to first destroy the AIDS viruses and, second, reconstitute the immune system.

Representative Henry Waxman, Chairman of the House Subcommittee on Health and Environment, has publicly stated that if a vaccine is found for AIDS, it will be in the late 1990's at the earliest.

WHAT WILL KILL THE AIDS VIRUS?

The real question is, "How long will the AIDS virus survive outside the body?"

The AIDS virus is a fairly fragile one. If it is placed in a hostile environment, its protective envelope will be broken and it will be killed fairly soon.   However, in a friendly environment, it can survive for months.   Almost all of the testing of the AIDS viruses has been in test tubes. Testing in real-life environments is another thing.

As we have pointed out, the AIDS virus will live for many months in liquid blood, and it can survive for seven days in dried blood or dried saliva.

We know that holding the AIDS virus at 60°C (140°F) for several hours will kill it. Chlorine or alcohol, in sufficient concentration, will kill it.   However, these solutions can not be applied to viruses inside the human body.

THE IMPACT OF THE FACTS

The "facts" can vary slightly, especially where projections must be made.   For example, in September, 1985, based on the privileged information available to him, Senator Orren Hatch, stated that 1,000,000 to 1,500,000 were infected with AIDS, (AIDS--STAGE 1).

The number of people in the U.S. with AIDS--STAGE 1 could already be as high as 3,000,000, according to the July, 1985 issue of LIFE.[13]

Opinions of respected researchers, medical authorities and scientists vary widely. In this chapter, we have tried to present just the factual information. We must now move on to investigate how these facts impact the U.S. and you personally.

Since AIDS is 100 percent fatal, since at present there seems to be little likelihood that a vaccine will be found for it, and since the 1 million or more in America who are presently infected with the disease--that is, have AIDS-STAGE 1--(most of whom do not know that they have it) are continuing to infect others today, a very large number of Americans could die of AIDS within the next ten to fifteen years.

3

THE EPIDEMIC OF AIDS

America is to the point of realizing that AIDS is an epidemic and, I believe, eventually will be called a pandemic or a plague.

On its July, 1985, cover, LIFE magazine had the following headline:

NOW NO ONE IS SAFE FROM AIDS

The August 5, 1985, TIME magazine had this headline:

AIDS: A SPREADING SCOURGE --INCURABLE AND LETHAL, THE DISEASE IS TAKING A MOUNTING TOLL

The cover headline of the August 12, 1985, issue of TIME was:

THE FRIGHTENING AIDS EPIDEMIC COMES OUT OF THE CLOSET

These are but a sampling of the headlines that point out the fact that the people of the United States are becoming very concerned about the epidemic proportions of AIDS.

AIDS evidently started in Central Africa. In the countries of that region of

Africa, AIDS is already in epidemic proportions and is still growing. Dr. Clymeck, a
tropical disease expert from Brussels, puts
the minimum figure of Africans infected with
AIDS at above 30 million. In Rwanda, one
out of five has AIDS and in Zaire, one out
of six.

Evidently it then spread to Haiti, and
there too it is in epidemic proportions. It
then came into the homosexual community in
the United States, where it is nearing epidemic proportions. It is just getting started
in the heterosexual community in America,
and this should be of concern to every citizen of the United States.

U.S. doctors first identified AIDS victims only four years ago, and there was only
a small number of cases, mostly in the
homosexual community. Today, there are
more than 14,000 people in the U.S. with
AIDS--STAGE 2, the number is doubling
every year, and the disease is reaching into
the heterosexual commmunity. Unlike the
bubonic plague, tuberculosis and other
plagues, AIDS seems to kill everyone it
infects.

THE AIDS EPIDEMIC IN AMERICA

According to Dr. Ward Cates, of the
U.S. Centers For Disease Control, the other
name for AIDS should be "fear." It could
become one of those infectious diseases that
change history.

AIDS is 100 percent fatal. There is no one who has had it more than four or five years who is alive today. If you read that AIDS has a 50-percent mortality rate, that simply means that half of the people who have AIDS--STAGE 2 have not died yet. Since AIDS has a two- to five-year incubation period (AIDS--STAGE 1), an infected person can infect numerous individuals before he even realizes that he has it.

As we mentioned in Chapter 1, Dr. James Curran, head of the Centers for Disease Control's Task Force on AIDS, says that sample studies based on blood tests suggest that 500,000 to 1,000,000 Americans have now been infected and are carriers of the AIDS virus. These are people whose symptoms have not yet appeared. They have AIDS--STAGE 1 and can infect others.

If this doubling of the number of cases each year (AIDS--STAGE 2) continues, and it could go up even more rapidly than that, this is what we would have across the coming years:

Table 3.1

YEAR		NUMBER OF CASES AIDS--STAGE 2
1985	=	14,000
1986	=	28,000
1987	=	56,000
1988	=	112,000
1989	=	224,000

1990	=	448,000
1991	=	896,000
1992	=	1,792,000
1993	=	3,584,000
1994	=	7,168,000
1995	=	14,336,000
1996	=	28,672,000
1997	=	57,344,000

This disease is becoming as much a heterosexual disease as a homosexual one. It has the potential of infecting much of the population. According to Mathilde Krim, a research biologist at the Memorial Sloan-Kettering Cancer Center in Manhattan, health authorities are concerned about the possible role of prostitutes in spreading the epidemic.

In earlier days, if a man got gonorrhea, the public health officials would find out the name of the woman from whom he contracted it. They would then ask her to give the names and addresses of her sexual partners and would contact them to get the names of their sexual partners. Frequently this could mount up to over 100 individuals involved. This was with a disease having an incubation period of just a few days. If the incubation period had been two to five years, as with AIDS, the number could have run into the thousands.

Following this thinking, it could be that any of those living a nonmonogamous sexual life-style could become infected before this epidemic of AIDS has run its course. What percentage of the population would you estimate lives in a nonmonogamous fashion?

20 TO 25 PERCENT OF THE U.S. POPULATION COULD DIE OF AIDS WITHIN THE NEXT TWELVE YEARS

As Table 3.1 showed, by 1997 we could have 50 million cases of AIDS. That would mean that roughly 25 percent of the population of the United States would die or be terminally ill within the next twelve years!

Don McAlvany, publisher of the acclaimed MCALVANY INTELLIGENCE ADVISOR and an acknowledged analyst of geopolitical trends, agrees that 20 to 25 percent of the U.S. population dying of AIDS is a reasonable estimate.[1]   R. E. McMaster, well-known analyst of sociological trends and cycles, author of some outstanding books, and editor of the newsletter THE REAPER, feels that 20 to 25 percent is low and that the death toll could become much higher.[2]

If this number of U.S. citizens die of AIDS within the next twelve years, then AIDS will certainly be classified as a history-changing plague. I would consider it far more than an epidemic. As we discussed earlier, in times past we have had such pandemics as the bubonic plague, the black death and the plagues of flu. Joining in the ranks of these other terrible plagues, I believe will be the AIDS plague.

THE FEAR OF AIDS SPREADS

Public opinion polls show that the fear of AIDS is spreading rapidly. We must ensure that this fear (legitimate fear) translates into productive action and not hysteria or panic. Typical of the polls was the one published by STAR magazine on September 24, 1985.[3]   They said that despite reassurances from public health authorities, more than 90 percent of women and 82 percent of men surveyed said they were worried about the spread of AIDS here. When asked to rate their concern on a scale of 1 to 10, the majority of women (55.2 percent) rated it at 10.

STAR magazine reported Dr. Mathilde Krim, chairperson of the board of trustees of the AIDS Medical Foundation, a research organization founded by scientists and physicians dealing with AIDS, as saying:

> "It is quite realistic for people to be concerned about AIDS spreading to the heterosexual community. With up to a million people having been infected so far, 8 to 10 million could be infected over the next 10 years. Not everybody infected with the virus comes down with AIDS, but they can become carriers."

The fact that a percentage of both adult and childhood cases of AIDS fit none of the known risk groups has helped to raise concern that the disease may be spreading to the general population.

The fear is real and the danger is real. It is time to recognize the danger and act-- act in a cool and collected way, but act we must.

IT IS TIME TO CALL
AN "AIDS RED ALERT"

The congress and the president of the United States have sworn to provide for the "general welfare." If they are going to fulfill this constitutional requirement, they must begin to take AIDS seriously and to enact legislation to protect the public. We will discuss what they should do later in this book. Here we are talking about their attitude, their priorities and their sense of urgency and responsibility.

The surgeon general of the United States is the individual with direct responsibility to ensure the health of the population in general. As of late 1985, he has been totally silent on the subject of AIDS. It is time that he break his silence and declare an "AIDS Red Alert" or a national "AIDS Emergency." How bad does the plague of AIDS have to get before he acts?

City councils and federal and local public health officials are not treating AIDS with the seriousness it deserves. They are more concerned about the civil rights of individuals here and there than the health and welfare of the vast majority of the public.

The EXECUTIVE INTELLIGENCE REVIEW (EIR) shares the concern and urgency of combating AIDS:[4]

More of the world's leading experts on AIDS have publicly joined with the growing number of specialists that are warning that AIDS could become a global catastrophe far worse than even full-scale thermonuclear war. In a series of exclusive interviews given to this magazine at the end of September, Belgian tropical-diseases expert Dr. Clymeck has put the minimum figure of Africans infected with AIDS, in the nine-nation so-called AIDS Belt, at above 30 million people. Both he and Dr. Sonigo of the Pasteur Institute's research team on AIDS, in independent interviews to EIR, stated that they would consider the "risk" population for AIDS in Africa to be the entire African population.

Additional world authorities on the subject of AIDS have confirmed to us the true, shocking dimensions of the global AIDS breakout. Dr. John Seale was, until the late 1970s, at the Veneral-Disease Division of St. Thomas-Middlesex Hospital. Dr. Seale asserted that in his assessment of the AIDS situation, "We are heading toward a world disaster." He stressed: "Complacency is the worst possible reaction!" Dr. Seale emphasized that his evaluation of the global threat of AIDS was not unique. "This Hazeltine of Harvard said AIDS may be the worst problem mankind has ever faced. And this young William Cates, of the CDC, talked about the potentialities of this for becoming a global disaster."

The National Democratic Policy Committee (NDPC) has published a report entitled:

AIDS IS MORE DEADLY
THAN NUCLEAR WAR

In it, they had this to say:[5]

At this very moment there is a major coverup being run on the real story of AIDS. AIDS is more deadly than nuclear war. Already the AIDS virus has infected tens of millions of Africans in at least nine different countries in the sub-Saharan area. The actual number of cases in the United States are orders of magnitude more than the so-called official statistics. Washington, in disregard for the general welfare of our people and our national security, is desperately trying to keep the lid on the real AIDS story. . . .
The real number of AIDS cases in this country and worldwide is far, far larger than what is being reported. AIDS is rampaging in epidemic form across Africa and tropical disease

experts report that, for example, a full 20% of the population of Rwanda is carrying the antibodies to AIDS, indicating, at minimum, that they have been exposed to the disease. In the United States, one of our nation's leading medical schools has publicly stated that the real number of AIDS victims may be ten times or more the "official" figure. . . .

One leading medical school on the West Coast has published a study which shows that the actual number of AIDS victims is from 3 to 10 times the CDC "official" statistics. That would mean that, in reality, at least 140,000 Americans may already be AIDS victims, and 14 million may be walking around with the antibodies indicating that they have been exposed to the disease.

We must begin right now to treat AIDS as a plague, a pandemic, and to think in terms of what we should do as a nation. As we will discuss later, the place to begin is by testing those in critical occupations (health care, child care, food handling, etc.) and only allowing those who test negative on the AA blood test to work in those occupations.

While we are waiting for the government to act, we must be concerned about how we as individuals can protect ourselves and our families, in order to minimize the possibility of acquiring AIDS.

4

HOW YOU CAN PROTECT YOURSELF

My motivation for writing this book is to help you and others. I want to help eliminate any panic in your heart. Most of all, I want to help you avoid getting AIDS.

There are a number of specific areas that you might want to consider when thinking about protecting yourself from getting AIDS. The primary areas are:

1. Blood transfusions

2. Sexual activity

3. Exchange of saliva

4. Introducing an AIDS virus into a mucous membrane or a scratch

We will discuss each of these areas one at a time and then give a summary list at the end of the chapter.

First, we need to keep in mind that you are not going to get AIDS from handshakes, toilet seats or handling an object that someone with AIDS has handled. Your skin is a protective shield against things like that. You are not going to get it if someone with AIDS sneezes in your vicinity out in public. You actually have to take someone else's body fluids into your own body to acquire AIDS.

AVOID GETTING AIDS THROUGH
BLOOD TRANSFUSIONS OR NEEDLES

It has definitely been proven that people have acquired AIDS by having blood transfusions with blood that contains the AIDS virus. With these people, the symptoms of AIDS--STAGE 2 appears the most rapidly.

One of the things we must realize is that the test for AIDS that the blood banks are using on blood does not 100 percent ensure that the blood does not contain AIDS viruses. It will eliminate most of the blood containing AIDS viruses, but there is no guarantee.

A safer way to go would be to have blood transfusions from your own family members, whom you know are free of AIDS. It would not hurt to have their blood types and yours checked ahead of time, so that you know who could and who could not give you blood.

One of the things that a number of people are doing is going in several times to donate their own blood to be stored in a segregated way, so that if they ever need a blood transfusion, because of an accident, an emergency or elective surgery, their own blood can be used. Many Hollywood stars are doing this, such as George Hamilton and John Matuszak. This is the safest way of all.

The October 18, 1985 issue of the excellent EXECUTIVE INTELLIGENCE REVIEW had this to say about our nation's blood supply:[1]

> There can be no more acute threat to a country's national security than the contamination of its blood supply with a deadly and highly contagious disease. Leading U.S. experts such as Dr. Myron Essex of the Harvard School of Public Health are now asserting that indeed America's blood supply, despite the precautions recently introduced, is still contaminated with the AIDS virus. But despite the evidence at hand, government health officials and the Atlanta Centers for Disease Control are maintaining their cover-up.
>
> At an extraordinary forum on AIDS on October 3, sponsored by the Harvard School of Public Health, Dr. Myron Essex, chairman of the Department of Cancer Biology, warned that in the next 5-10 years, 4 to 5 million Americans could be infected with the AIDS virus. Dr. Essex declared: "We need to act fast if those numbers are not to be 40 million to 50 million Americans infected and 4 million to 5 million with AIDS outright." Dr. Essex further emphasized that, despite reassuring statements to the contrary from the Red Cross and other agencies, "unfortunately, our blood supply is not safe."

The Harvard forum was titled, "Can AIDS Be Stopped?" and was opened with remarks by Harvey V. Fineberg; dean of the Harvard School of Public Health.

Dr. Essex asserted that it was "a gross exaggeration" to imply, as national public-health officials have done, that the "blood supply is now fully safe. I don't believe that. The blood supply is safer than it was a year ago, but it would be totally misleading to have people think the blood supply is safe. If I were considering the possibliity of elective surgery, I would donate my own blood in advance." Dr. Essex added that, although tests might detect 95% of the contaminated blood samples, in the actual setting of a blood bank, "it's extremely unlikely that the test is picking up more than 90%, and my guess is it's 75-80%. I'd be shocked if it's any better than that."

Because of the poverty in Africa, the same needle is used on many patients. AIDS has been spread there in that manner. Of course you would want to avoid having a needle used on you that has ever been used on anyone else. As we said earlier, the use of a common needle is the reason many drug users have acquired AIDS. The amount of blood dried on a needle is miniscule, but that is all it takes to get AIDS.

AIDS FROM SEXUAL ACTIVITY

As mentioned previously, either homo-sexual or heterosexual individuals can acquire AIDS through the exchange of body fluids during sexual activity.

Heterosexual men can transmit AIDS to women through the injection of their semen. The vagina, being a major mucous membrane in the body, will readily play host to many kinds of viruses, and certainly the AIDS virus would find an ideal home there. According to GOOD HOUSEKEEPING (November, 1985), well over one hundred women have contracted AIDS sexually from their husbands or lovers.[2]

Men can acquire AIDS through having sex with women in the same way that they acquire gonorrhea, syphilis and other sexually transmitted diseases through intercourse. Because men can acquire AIDS from prostitutes, all military personnel are being tested. Most likely, the AIDS virus enters the opening in the penis, where it again finds a place in which it can reside and begin to multiply.

When the AIDS virus is introduced into a mucous membrane, it develops more slowly than when introduced directly into the bloodstream. One of the reasons that AIDS has spread rapidly among homosexuals is because of anal intercourse. In anal intercourse, often some of the tiny capillaries are ruptured and this gives the AIDS virus a direct entry into the bloodstream. Herpes lesions in the vagina would also allow easier absorption of ejaculation fluid containing the AIDS virus.

The way to protect yourself from acquiring AIDS through sexual activity is to first know that your marriage partner is faithful and does not have AIDS, and then remain sexually faithful to that partner. The use of condoms can help reduce the spread of AIDS, but remember that condoms can break or slip off.

Even if your partner had sex with someone as much as five years ago, he or she could have AIDS and not know it. Thus, truthfulness between marriage partners about past sexual activity is going to be essential. If there is any doubt, be tested. If there is any likelihood of either partner having AIDS, the AA blood test would be in order.

Once it is known that both parties are AIDS free, then it is absolutely essential to live a monogamous sexual life. This is being recognized not only by Christian ministers and teachers, but also by those in secular and government organizations. The following came across the national wire services August 14, 1985:

> A top scientific expert on AIDS says the best way to stop the spread of the deadly disease is for the government to persuade Americans to develop socially responsible sexual behavior. Doctor James Mason of the Centers for

Disease Control says (on ABC) that means monogamous relationships.

As we have seen, AIDS is not just a homosexual disease, but it can strike anyone, especially those with more than one sexual partner (in the last five years). As time goes by, it may well not be enough to take the word of your potential marriage partner about his or her past sexual activity. Individuals are going to want to know more about past experiences in detail and perhaps even to take AA blood tests. The excellent magazine, GOOD HOUSEKEEPING, is rightfully concerned about the ladies who comprise its readership. It had this to say on the subject:[2]

> If [a] woman has been in a relationship that has been completely monogamous on both sides for the past five years or so, she has nothing to worry about.
> But if she or her partner strays ouside the relationship, the window of risk begins to open. The same is true of a single woman with more than one sexual partner.

People will want to know that the individual they are marrying is AIDS-free. One of the better ways to ensure this is to marry a virgin. I forecast that the premium on marrying virgins will rise to the point that it will be the vogue and almost essen-

tial by 1996.   We will discuss this further
later.

PROTECTION FROM ACQUIRING AIDS
BY AN EXCHANGE OF SALIVA

We normally would think of the
exchange of saliva as occurring in deep,
passionate kissing, and this is the major way
that someone else's saliva might enter your
body.   However, there are many other ways
that saliva can be exchanged.   One obvious
way is by giving direct mouth-to-mouth
resuscitation to someone who has drowned.
Firemen and paramedics will no longer do
this.   They now have a plastic device that
they put over the person's mouth, which has
a tube about ½ inch in diameter that the
rescuer can place in his mouth.   If firemen
and paramedics are this concerned about
acquiring AIDS through mouth-to-mouth
resuscitation, this should cause the general
public to be equally concerned about
acquiring AIDS through contact with someone
else's saliva.   Until it is absolutely
100-percent proven that AIDS cannot be
acquired this way, assume that it is a way
to acquire AIDS.

If you have a swimming pool and even a
remote possibility of having to give mouth-
to-mouth resuscitation to a casual acquain-
tance, you may want to purchase one of the
mouth-to-mouth resuscitation devices, called
"pocket masks," to keep handy.   You may
also want to take one of these along on any

outings to a lake.   They fold and you can
carry one in your pocket.   These can be
purchased for about $10 each at your local
medical supply store.   If they don't have
them in stock, they can order some from the
manufacturer:

S. L. O. Health Products, Inc.
1155 Fifth Street
Los Osos, CA 93402
(805) 528-3197

There are other ways that an exchange
of saliva could occur.   For example, if you
were to drink from a glass or a bottle immediately after someone else, you could ingest
some of his saliva.   This is not likely, but
it is possible.

This brings us to the next point, which
is educating your children about the risk of
saliva exchange.   I know that this might
sound Victorian and puritanical, but we must
face facts as we know them.   Suppose your
youngster kisses one other person and that
kissing partner had only kissed one other
individual (within the last five years), and
yet that individual had kissed two other
individuals, each of whom had kissed two,
and so on, multiplied out much like a chain
letter.   In a sense, through that single kiss,
your child could be coming into contact with
hundreds or thousands of people.   Somewhere
in that chain, there could easily have been
someone with AIDS, unknowingly passing it
on to others.

I realize that, when I was in high school, if someone had told us not to "french kiss," I would have protested loudly. I certainly would have felt that it was curtailing my social life and probably would not have listened.

It is likely that many teenagers will disdain this advice, like they disdain advice on smoking and drugs. Therefore, at some point in the future, your children could unknowingly become infected with AIDS, just by a simple act of kissing.

It is possible that the morality of a hundred or two hundred years ago may come back. Then, one did not even kiss a date, except for a peck on the cheek, until the two were engaged and ready to be married.

The bottom line is that scientists have cautioned us about the exchange of saliva and, if we want to minimize the likelihood of acquiring AIDS, we need to avoid ingesting anyone else's saliva by any method, with the exception of our marriage partner.

AVOID INTRODUCING AN AIDS VIRUS INTO A MUCOUS MEMBRANE OR A SCRATCH

We know that the AIDS virus can live outside the body. As we said earlier, researchers have not yet determined how long it can live outside the body under all circumstances.

We also know that holding the AIDS virus at 60°C (140°F) for hours will kill the virus, as will concentrated chlorine or alcohol.   Researchers have not yet determined what other things will kill the virus.

The AIDS virus may be contained in someone's blood, saliva or tears, and we must take caution not to allow any of those body fluids from another individual to enter our body.   They could enter through one of our mucous membranes (mouth, eyes, nose or private openings) or an opening in our skin (cut, scratch, open sore and so forth).

If you have a scratch or an opening in your skin, you would want to avoid getting anyone else's blood, saliva or body fluids into that opening, because it would be a possible way to introduce the AIDS virus into your body.   For example, if in trying to help an automobile accident victim, you scratched your hand and then got his blood on your hands, this could give the AIDS virus an opportunity to enter your bloodstream.

It is also wise not to share a toothbrush or a razor with anyone, since these can expose you to minute quantities of blood.

You would also want to avoid drinking out of the same glass as someone else. Because of this concern, many churches formerly using a common cup for communion have gone to individual cups.

Because children with AIDS are not identified in schools or preschools, Oregon state gives this advice to teachers and others who may be required to give first aid to children:[3]

Wear disposable plastic gloves, if you have cuts, scratches, or other lesions on your hands, when providing first aid for bleeding injuries.

If you do not have hand lesions, gloves are not necessary, but you should wash your hands immediately after completing the first aid.

Avoid getting blood from an injured child in your mouth or eyes. If such an experience occurs, rinse the eye or mouth thoroughly with water.

Clean up any spilled blood with soap and water, followed by disinfection with a freshly-made solution of one part bleach to 10 parts water or 70% ethyl alcohol.

Dispose of blood-contaminated items in a plastic bag.

What if a curious child were to go over and stick his finger in a small puddle of blood during an emergency? What if he then stuck his finger in his mouth?

If you have someone with AIDS (STAGE 1 or 2) living with you, then additional precautions need to be taken. During Rock Hudson's last days, a great deal was done by the housekeeping staff to keep his Beverly Hills mansion free of germs. His staff would not allow entrance to anyone who had even a sniffle. They also did all they could to ensure that AIDS viruses from Rock were not spread to others. They continually wiped down everything with strong antiseptic. Any

silverware or china that Rock used was
sterilized, using the type of sterilizer used
in hospitals.

Hospitals are becoming very cautious in
handling AIDS patients. One hospital
recently circulated these precautions:[4]

1. Use gloves for contact with gross
body secretions and blood, such as
starting IV's, drawing blood including
both needle aspirations and through stop
cocks, dressing changes, emptying urine
collection bags, cleaning up spills, etc.

2. Needle disposal in puncture-proof
containers without breaking or recapping
needle. Needle box should be in the
room.

3. Laundry should be handled as isolation laundry, i.e., in plastic water-
soluble bags inside cloth isolation
laundry bags.

4. Waste should be disposed of in the
same manner as all isolation waste,
i.e., in double red bags which are then
placed in isolation garbage cans.

5. Disposable dishes will be used for
serving meals, etc.

6. All specimens must be labeled
"Blood and Body Fluid Precautions" and
double bagged out of the patient's room
for transport to Lab. Lab slips must
also be labeled "Blood and Body Fluid
Precautions" and attached to the outside
of the double bag.

7.   Spills of blood and other body secretions should be cleaned up promptly by a gloved employe with a solution of 5.25% sodium hypochlorite (household bleach) diluted 1:10 with water.

8.   Showers and tubs should be decontaminated daily with 1:10 solution of 5.25% sodium hypochlorite and water by housekeeping.

9.   Respiratory Therapy ventilator tubing may be pasteurized. Any instrument that comes into contact with blood or other secretions must be sterilized before reuse. Lensed instruments must be sterilized.

10.   Clinitron beds should not be used for AIDS or suspected AIDS patients because of the extreme difficulty in decontaminating them adequately.

Notice item 5: hospitals using disposable dishes for AIDS patients. They recognize the potent danger that exists in AIDS-laden saliva.

We also have the problem of the AIDS virus in tears. The primary way that this could affect you is through food handlers. As we pointed out earlier, if a food handler with AIDS wiped a tear from his eye or stuck his finger in his mouth and then handled some bread which absorbed the fluid, and a few minutes later you ate that bread, it would be just as though he had put that tear or that saliva on the end of your tongue.

Right now some restaurant owners require food handlers to have a turberculin test to be sure they are not spreading that disease. Already, some restaurants are requiring all their food handlers to take the AIDS Antibody (AA) blood test. At the ENSERCH Company in Dallas, Texas, after giving all of their food handlers the AA test, those who tested positive were removed from their positions. We discuss requiring the AA blood test and an AIDS health card in Chapter 6. This health card would have to have an expiration date, much like a driver's license.

Concern of getting AIDS from food handlers will probably not be high on your list of concerns at this point in time, but as the AIDS epidemic multiplies, and tens of thousands, then hundreds of thousands, and then millions of people per year contract AIDS, at some point many of these precautions may become mandatory for your safety. This would be especially true if restaurants do not test their employees with the AA blood test.

Another area where the AIDS virus in tears could be of concern is in eye examinations, especially when contact lenses are used. Since scientists at the National Institutes of Health found the AIDS virus in tears, the Centers for Disease Control published these guidelines to help prevent the transmission of the AIDS virus via tears:[5]

1. Health care professionals performing eye examinations or other procedures involving contact with tears should wash their hands immediately after a procedure and between patients. Handwashing alone should be sufficient, but when practical and convenient, disposable gloves may be worn. The use of gloves is advisable when there are cuts, scratches or dermatologic lesions on the hands. Use of other protective measures, such as masks, goggles, or gowns, is not indicated.

2. Instruments that come into direct contact with external surfaces of the eye should be wiped clean and then disinfected by: (a) a 5- to 10-minute exposure to a fresh solution of 3% hydrogen peroxide; or (b) a fresh solution containing 5,000 parts per million (mg/L) free available chlorine--a 1/10 dilution of common household bleach (sodium hypochlorite); or (c) 70% ethanol; or (d) 70% isopropanol. The device should be thoroughly rinsed in tap water and dried before reuse.

3. Contact lenses used in trial fittings should be disinfected between each fitting by one of the following regimens:
      a. Disinfection of trial hard lenses with a commercially available hydrogen peroxide contact lens disinfecting system currently approved for soft contact lenses.

(Other hydrogen peroxide preparations may contain preservatives that could discolor the lenses.) Alternatively, most trial hard lenses can be treated with a standard heat disinfection regimen used for soft lenses (78-80 C [172-176 F] for 10 minutes). Practitioners should check with hard lens suppliers to ascertain which lenses can be safely heat-treated.

b. Rigid gas permeable (RGP) trial fitting lenses can be disinfected using the above hydrogen peroxide disinfection system. RGP lenses may warp if they are heat-disinfected.

c. Soft trial fitting lenses can be disinfected using the same hydrogen peroxide system. Some soft lenses have also been approved for heat disinfection.

Other than hydrogen peroxide, the chemical disinfectants used in standard contact lens solutions have not yet been tested for their activity against HTLV-III/LAV. Until other disinfectants are shown to be suitable for disinfecting HTLV-III/LAV, contact lenses used in the eyes of patients suspected or known to be infected with HTLV-III/LAV are most safely handled by hydrogen peroxide disinfection.

AIDS AND PREGNANCY

If you are planning to have a child, you and your spouse should get an AA blood test before you become pregnant. If either test is positive, which means you have AIDS--STAGE 1, do not get pregnant.

If, for some reason, you are considering artificial insemination, be sure that the semen donor has had the AA blood test and that the result was negative. If you cannot be assured of that, you should wait until a donor is found who has shown negative on the test.

A SUMMARY LIST OF THINGS TO DO TO PROTECT YOURSELF FROM AIDS:

1. Avoid sex with anyone but your own marriage partner.

2. Avoid even an exchange of saliva, except with your marriage partner.

3. Educate your children concerning the risk of saliva exchange and other hazards.

4. Give direct mouth-to-mouth resuscitation only to those you know are clean. Use a mouth-to-mouth resuscitation device with all others.

5. Don't drink from the same glass or bottle as anyone else, unless you are positive that individual is free of AIDS.

6. Store your own blood.

7. Avoid blood transfusions, except from family members, or from your own stored blood.

8. Do not allow a needle to be used on you that has been used on anyone else.

9. Do not share a toothbrush.

10. Do not share a razor.

11. Exercise careful hygiene in public restrooms.

12. If you are a dentist, paramedic, prison guard or have an occupation that brings you into contact with the body fluids of others, wear rubber gloves and other protective attire.

13. Women with positive results on the AIDS Antibody (AA) blood test should avoid getting pregnant.

14. Women planning on artificial insemination should be sure the semen donor has had the AIDS Antibody test and was shown negative.

15. Both parties should be tested for the Aids Antibody before getting married.

Some of the above precautions may ultimately be proven unnecessary, but until the surgeon general or some other major medical authority comes out with a clear statement that the AIDS virus cannot be transferred by an exchange of saliva or by ingesting the tears of an AIDS-infected individual, then you will be far better off to be safe than sorry.

This may mean somewhat of a change of life-style for you and your children, but the change, and any inconvenience now, could be well worth it to help you and your family avoid getting AIDS.

5
THE EFFECT OF AIDS
ON THE ECONOMY

As we begin to look at the effect of AIDS on the economy, we will be considering what effect the decrease by 20 or 25 percent of the U.S. population would have on the economy and on certain industries. If AIDS proves to be the history-changing plague that we believe it will be, this is an area that needs our careful consideration, since we all live in an economic world--that is, we get paid, we make purchases and so forth.

If 20 to 25 percent of the population dies, for example, there could be a surplus of houses and office and industrial buildings. Therefore, real estate investments could do poorly as the plague progresses.

There will also be a significant impact on other industries and occupations.

THE IMPACT OF AIDS
ON INSURANCE COMPANIES

The medical expenses of an AIDS victim average $145,000-150,000. The insurance companies can handle a few of these, but there is not enough money in the health insurance companies to handle 50 million

Americans at over $145,000 each. At some point in time, they will have to declare bankruptcy, cease to give medical care to AIDS victims or the government will have to take over and care for the AIDS victims.

As people change jobs, it may be that, in order to get hospitalization insurance at the new job, they will have to test negative on the AA blood test. Thus, we could see less changing of jobs.

Some insurance companies are now offering "AIDS insurance" to those without symptoms.

Life insurance companies could be in trouble. The premiums on their life insurance policies are based on what they call "mortality tables." These are tables giving the average life expectancy of men and women at each age. However, if all of a sudden 20 to 25 percent of their policy holders die, say an average of twenty to thirty years before the insurance companies were expecting it, these insurance companies might not be able to pay off all of those death benefit claims.

Life insurance companies are already using the HTLV-III antibody (AA) blood test. The WALL STREET JOURNAL reported the following on October 18, 1985:[1]

> On Oct. 1, Home Office Reference Laboratory, a Shawnee Mission, Kan., lab that tests blood and urine samples for about 1,000 life-insurance com-

panies, began running a series of tests for exposure to the HTLV-3 virus that is presumed to cause AIDS.

The lab, a subsidiary of Business Men's Assurance Co. of Kansas City, Mo., is performing the tests for about 25 life-insurance companies, according to Ken Stelzer, the lab's president. He says 300 to 500 blood samples were tested in the first two weeks.

A positive finding indicates that a person has AIDS antibodies in his blood and therefore has been exposed to the virus. It doesn't indicate that he has AIDS or will get it. But researchers believe that his chances of developing AIDS within five years are between 5% and 20%. Because the disease is invariably fatal, insurers tend to consider anyone with AIDS antibodies an unacceptable risk. The CDC believes that as many as one million Americans have been so exposed.

Life insurers are among the first businesses (other than blood banks guarding the safety of blood products) to make much use of AIDS-antibody tests. Others would like to.

I would counsel both health insurance and life insurance companies to begin to look at AIDS very seriously, and to do whatever they can to prepare for the tremendous impact that it is going to have on their financial reserves. Of necessity, they will

need to use the AA blood test on all new
applicants.

If the AIDS epidemic goes as I believe it
will, then ultimately individuals are going to
need to be prepared not to receive all the
insurance benefits that they are anticipating.
I certainly hope that this does not come
true, but if we look at the numbers
realistically, this is what the future seems
to hold.

THE IMPACT OF AIDS ON HOSPITALS

At one time I lived on Catalina Island.
Avalon, the only town on the island, had
1,500 people and a ten-bed hospital. Thus,
the community was anticipating that no more
than a small percentage of the people would
ever need hospitalization at any one time.
If all of a sudden 20 percent of the people
had needed to be hospitalized, which would
have been 300 people, that little ten-bed
hospital would have been far from adequate.
If the AIDS epidemic proceeds as I believe it
will, our hospitals are going to be flooded
with AIDS patients and there will not be
nearly enough room for all of them to be
admitted.

One AIDS victim complained that he had
"no place to go and die." The hospitals
could not keep him and, without an income
or other resources, he really did not have a
place to go. Perhaps in the future there
will be a type of nursing home or hospital
that is devoted exclusively to terminal AIDS

patients that will give people with AIDS a place to go and die gracefully. This could be a service that churches could provide, just as they have built orphanages and homes for the elderly.

I suspect that the government will ultimately be forced to step in and convert unused military bases into AIDS camps or AIDS retirement villages. The private sector will simply be unable to handle the coming AIDS tidal wave.

THE IMPACT OF AIDS
ON RESTAURANTS

We have already talked about the possibility of body fluids of an AIDS-infected food handler being transferred to food and then eaten by a restaurant patron. We mentioned that the Abilene Medical Center in Abilene, Texas had all of its food handlers tested with the AA blood test and terminated one who tested positive, because of its concern about AIDS being spread through food.

If this fear becomes widespread, and if it is a justified fear, then all restaurants will be forced to give all of their people AA blood tests, more often than annually, or the number of people eating out will drop dramatically. This likely could include even the fast food chains.

One certainly would not want to be holding stock in restaurants and fast food chains five or ten years from now, because many of them could go bankrupt.

THE IMPACT OF AIDS ON SCHOOLS

As we will see in a forthcoming chapter, it is possible that the future of schools will resemble something like this: a teacher in a room with a video camera and all the students in their homes or isolated study cells receiving the material on television sets (video monitors), without having a great deal of body contact with the other students.

If this scenario comes true, the tax burden on communities, both to maintain the existing school buildings, which would be largely unused, and to purchase all the necessary video equipment, could be a real strain and certainly would have an economic impact on the community.

BUSINESSES THAT WILL BE HELPED BY AIDS

Up until now, we have only talked about industries that might potentially be hurt by the AIDS epidemic. There are also a number of businesses and industries which may be helped by the AIDS plague.

We have already mentioned that hospitals will be helped, since they can almost be guaranteed 100 percent occupancy--that is, as long as the health insurance companies or the government can pay for the care of the AIDS victims.

Another industry that will be helped will be that of morticians. In any plague, as the number of casualties grows, morticians begin to work night and day to care for all of the deceased. Not only will the funeral homes be in high demand but also the products that they use.

Companies that build caskets and provide headstones for graves will be working multiple shifts to keep up with the demand. Similarly, cemetary plots could be at a premium. The law of supply and demand says that the prices for these will rise, as the prices for caskets and mortician services continue to rise. (You might consider pre-paying your funeral and burial expenses now.)

Another industry that will do very well is the companies that make the HTLV-III Antibody (AA) blood test. One such company is called Electro-Nucleonics, Inc., whose OTC symbol is ENUC. They are rated as a B minus stock by Standard and Poors and have been in business since 1971. They are located in Fairfield, New Jersey (201/227-6700). They make medical diagnostic systems and equipment, including disposable diagnostic supplies.

In March, 1985 the federal government licensed them to produce and distribute the blood test which tests for the HTLV-III antibody. It is estimated that they will sell at least 70 million of these each year. They shipped 150,000 of them in March, 1985 alone. This AIDS Antibody blood test (in addition to the ongoing diagnostic systems and chemical labs that they supply worldwide) could give a boost to this stock. At present, this company is one of only three licensed to make the AIDS blood test. The other two companies are:

. Abbott Laboratories
Litton Bionetics

Investing in these stocks would be a speculative investment. We all wish that AIDS were not here and that people did not have to manufacture these blood tests, but looking at life as it exists rather than as we would wish it, these companies should fare well as the AIDS epidemic runs its course.

Moving on to occupations that may be helped by the AIDS plague, it may be that teachers, child care workers, health care personnel (doctors, nurses, etc.) and such will come to be in demand, because they might come to be known as "hazardous duties."

This is not meant to be an exhaustive list of types of businesses and occupations that the AIDS plague will help. These are simply a few. A little careful contemplation will bring to mind other industries and companies that will do well during an AIDS epidemic.

AIDS AND THE QUESTION OF DEFLATION VERSUS INFLATION

One of the most important questions facing the investor is whether the future will bring deflation (prices dropping) or continued inflation.

With the advent of the AIDS plague, something new and powerful has entered the debate. Before we get into how AIDS could bring about deflation or inflation, we need to review the law of supply and demand.

The law of supply and demand controls the price of anything, whether it be a share of IBM stock, a gallon of gasoline, or a bushel of tomatoes. If there is more supply than there is demand, the price will fall until it comes into an equilibrium. As the price falls, people become more interested in buying and, thus, it will fall to a price at which the supply and demand come into balance. On the other hand, if the demand is greater than the supply, the price will continue to rise until fewer and fewer people are able to afford it, and then an equilibrium will be established between supply/demand and price.

If someone asks me why the price of a stock or of gold, silver or some other entity is going up or down, I tell him that it is because of supply and demand, and that is the **only** reason. All of the other things that people discuss are simply reasons why the supply or the demand may be rising or declining.

For example, if a major war were to break out someplace and many people rushed to buy gold, the demand would be increasing while the supply remained steady. Thus, the price would have to go up. It is really

the law of supply and demand that causes
the price to rise. In this case, the war is
simply the factor that would cause the
demand to increase.

When I first began to analyze the
impact of AIDS on the economy, I thought it
would be deflationary. My reasoning was
that if 20 percent of the U.S. population
were to disappear tomorrow, the supply
would remain the same and the demand
would shrink by 20 percent. I then asked
what would happen to prices if the demand
were to shrink that much with the supply
remaining constant. Under those conditions,
prices would fall.

However, there was a flaw in that
logic, as I examined it further. The supply
would NOT remain constant. As I said in
Chapter 1:

After 1400, the black death
returned many times to plague Europe,
until about 1700. The black death
hastened the breakup of medieval
society. Agriculture came to a near
standstill. The production of goods
fell. Goods became scarce and, thus,
prices rose.

Because laborers were scarce,
wages rose. This caused revolts to
break out in England, France, and
elsewhere. This pandemic led to hysteria.

In the wake of the black death, there
was inflation, because the plague shrank the

supply faster than it did the demand. With AIDS, all of those in STAGE 2 (and there will eventually be millions) will still be consuming but will not be producing. They will not simply disappear, as I first thought. Instead, they will be requiring goods and services, so the demand will remain high, while the supply dwindles. This is just the first way that AIDS could be inflationary.

As the AIDS epidemic progresses, the government will be spending billions to care for AIDS patients, which is the second way that AIDS could be inflationary. At present, AIDS--STAGE 2 victims receive Social Security benefits. Later, the government may even have to house and care for the millions of terminally ill AIDS victims. Also, the government will not have the tax revenues that would have come in from these AIDS victims, had they lived and continued to work. This will make our federal deficit even greater. This too will add fuel to the inflationary fires.

So it seems possible that AIDS will simply add to the other inflationary pressures. The government is going to have less income, which would be inflationary.

SUMMARY AND CONCLUSION

We have seen that AIDS could potentially add to the inflationary pressures. With 20 to 25 percent of the U.S. population possibly dying within the next twelve to fifteen years, this could rapidly decrease the supply of both goods and services.

There are some fields, such as morticians and hospitals, whose services will be in tremendous demand during the next ten years. This is unfortunate and we wish it were not so, but it seems to be likely.

We have seen that health insurance and life insurance companies could be in financial difficulty, if the AIDS epidemic progresses as we forecast. They will simply not have the financial resources to pay all of the claims that people will be making on them.

Restaurants and fast food chains are likely to be hit hard when the AIDS panic begins. Panic never does any good, but deep and urgent concern does. However, understanding mob psychology and mass hysteria, I foresee that at some point panic may set in and totally drive out of business many places that serve food.

However it turns out, AIDS is going to have a major impact on our economy, and the implications of this have yet to register in the mass media or in the minds of most of the population.

6
SHOULD THOSE WITH AIDS BE ISOLATED?

Before we examine the question, "Should those with AIDS be isolated?", we need to look at quarantining and what it means and at a bit of the background of quarantining. Quarantine is not a dirty word. The definition of a "quarantine" is:

An enforced isolation designed to prevent the spread of disease.

Quarantining can apply to animals, plants, or human beings. We have seen the quarantining of fruit that was coming out of areas in California where the Mediterranean fruit fly was discovered. This is a geographic quarantine, which is usually applied at points of entry and exit of a particular geographic region.

Governments also impose quarantines on ships, planes, and service carriers. This type of quarantining began in Western Europe during the 1300's for protection against the bubonic plague, which could be carried on ships trading with Asia. Governments today impose quarantines on exotic animals being brought into the country. They also require fumigation of cargoes against insects and so forth.

Governments also quarantine individuals at times. This practice goes far back to biblical days. For example, concerning leprosy, we read the following in the Old Testament book of Leviticus:

> 29   "Now if a man or woman has an infection on the head or on the beard,
> 30   then the priest shall look at the infection, and if it appears to be deeper than his skin, and there is thin yellowish hair in it, then the priest shall pronounce him unclean; it is a scale, it is leprosy of the head or of the beard.
> 31   "But if the priest looks at the infection of the scale, and indeed, it appears to be no deeper than the skin, and there is no black hair in it, then the priest shall isolate the person with the scaly infection for seven days. . .
>
> 45   "As for the leper who has the infection, his clothes shall be torn, and the hair of his head shall be uncovered, and he shall cover his mustache and cry, 'Unclean! Unclean!'
> 46   He shall remain unclean all the days during which he has the infection; he is unclean. He shall live alone; his dwelling shall be outside the camp."
>
> --Leviticus 13

As can be seen here, if a person had a disease that was considered infectious, he was isolated. In some cases, he had to live away from the camp all by himself. Some people today would scream that their civil rights were being violated, but in God's Old Testament law, He evidently considered the well-being of the many more important than the civil rights of the few.

QUARANTINE IN THE
U.S.A. AND CANADA

When I was a boy, I had chicken pox, and I remember the public health officials coming out and tacking a quarantine sign on our house. They then came back a week or two later to be sure that I was well, and they took down the sign.

Along with vaccination, the quarantining of individuals was one way that smallpox has been virtually stamped out of the world.

My wife's mother, Mrs. Ruth Patterson, gives this account of the quarantine of her sister in Canada in 1940:

My sister had polio back in 1940 or whenever that really horrible year was when it was so bad. My mother nursed her in the bunkhouse, the rest of us did the work part in the house, all through that summer and fall, harvest and all the rest. It rained quite a lot, too, seemingly, especially when we were trying to boil up the dishes or all the bed linens from the isolation effort. We had an old burner set up in the backyard, sort of midway between the house and the bunkhouse, and we took their meals to them in the big canner, left it on the step of the bunkhouse, and mother washed the dishes first, then put them in the canner and we covered it and took it to the stove, first putting a lot of water in it. There was a lot of water carrying, also wood chopping that year, too, as that stove had to go pretty steadily some days. Dad did the disposal of all their wastes by digging holes and burying same. Also, he was the only one allowed off the property; the rest of us were in quarantine, until such time as the doctor said we were out.

Anyway, she is a mighty fine sister to still have around. She has a great courage, maybe greater than we will ever know. I remember I asked Mom one time when she came "out" to talk to us how she could stand "it," and if she wasn't scared sometimes and cried, 'cause I had to. Mom always told us that she was the same and she was very brave, so I guess I thought she couldn't be crying on the inside, if she was so very brave. Mom also told me that they did a lot of praying together. As she couldn't for a long time lift a finger to wipe away the tears or blow her nose or things like that, I guess there was a lot of ignoring the wet spots, as they had months together in that bunkhouse, before we were allowed to bring her into the house again. Mother never let her sit up at all those early days, but kept her wrapped warmly, and rolled her to move her.

In our consideration of past epidemics and quarantines, let's read what Dr. Debra Freeman said in an interview with Warren Hamerman of EXECUTIVE INTELLIGENCE REVIEW:[1]

If you follow the route of various epidemics, particularly the epidemics we've seen just in the course of the past century, the U.S. government in the past really distinguished itself in the field of public health. It always moved quickly, very quickly, with prophylactic measures. Of course, during the great tuberculosis epidemics, themselves born out of an economic breakdown in the United States, and also a large population with depressed immune systems among people who came over as immigrants under poor conditions, the country moved very rapidly. People were screened, of course, and if they showed positive on TB tests, they were placed in institutions where they could be treated, the sanitariums that most people are familiar with.

The interesting thing, though, was that when we were dealing with the TB epidemic, the first people who were quarantined were of course those who were showing acute symptoms of tuberculosis, but very quickly we moved toward a policy where anyone who screened positive on the tests being used, were moved to sanitariums. . . .

You had a similar situation with polio, which frankly was rather a small epidemic. It actually, I think, killed 57,000 people and affected 500,000 others between 1915 and 1955, when the Salk vaccine was introduced. Yet, despite the fact that in terms of the numbers, it was not that great—certainly nowhere near the magnitude of the current AIDS epidemic—the government moved quickly. We are not sure, for instance, that the virus was transmitted by insects, but because there was reason enough to believe so, during the course of the 1940s towns were sprayed with DDT in an effort to kill flies that might be infected. On the theory that polio was a summer disease, many towns delayed school openings. And in Milwaukee in 1944, a citywide quarantine was called preventing children from leaving their homes.

Some of these measures were effective in fact. Some of them turned out to not really address the cause of the disease. The important thing though was that in the field of public health, the government moved very quickly to take whatever prophylactic measures it could to protect its population. And the key to public health has always been prevention. This is exactly what we are ignoring in the current circumstances of AIDS.

In public health circles, there are said to be two basic ways to prevent the spread of communicable disease. One is by prevention and the other is through the quarantine of infected individuals. The second half of this--the quarantine of infected individuals--has almost become lost in recent years. When is the last time that you saw a quarantine sign on a house? The chances are that you have not seen one for a long, long time, if ever. But that was part of our American heritage and, in a way, part of our public health protection.

With past diseases in the United States, the quarantine lasted a week or two, or sometimes a few months, at the most. However, as we look at the possibility of quarantining or isolating AIDS victims, we would have to consider a quarantine that would last for years, which is infeasible, in some respects, since over 1 million Americans and their families would have to be isolated. The historical exception to past quarantines being of short duration was the leper colonies, where people spent the rest of their lives. Already there have been suggestions from some quarters to have "AIDS colonies."

Since total quarantining, in the tradi-
tional sense, is not likely to happen, we
need to examine what can be done to stop
the spread of this dreaded disease. If we
are to stop it, we must first identify the
people carrying AIDS and isolate them suf-
ficiently, so they do not spread the disease
to healthy people.

THE PLACE TO BEGIN
IS IDENTIFICATION

The Army is now giving AA blood tests
to recruits, and to all existing military personnel, to be sure that they do not have
AIDS. What is legitimate for the army to
do should be legitimate for other organizations.   Thus, we could potentially see
schools requiring students to have this blood
test each year, before they are allowed to
come to school.

This is not unthinkable--they will not
allow children to come to school unless they
have had their shots. If children have
chicken pox or even lice in their hair, they
are not allowed in schools. If they are
prevented from attending because of these
minor diseases, it may be that the public
will demand that the students with a major
disease, like AIDS, also be isolated.

A number of years ago, food handlers
were required to take a test for tuberculosis
before they were allowed to handle food.
Very likely, the requirement to have a blood
test for AIDS will be instituted, at some

point, for food handlers in both private restaurants and public eating places, such as schools, military bases and so forth.

In the studied opinion of knowledgeable medical authorities, all of those with physical contact with the public should be required to take the AA blood test. This would include occupation such as:

    Health care workers
    Day care workers
    Food handlers, processors and pickers
    Barbers and beauticians
    School teachers
    Blood bank employees

If they tested positive, these authorities feel that they should not be allowed to work in these areas. This would be a minimum place to start. However, even more desirable would be to have everyone tested, not just those in critical occupations.

A NATIONAL BLOOD TEST?

In a cryotech laboratory, there is a sign that says:

    "GET YOUR BLOOD TEST.
     NO TEST--NO PAY."

That indeed may wind up being the sign of the future.

One possibility is to require all U.S. residents, citizens as well as legal and illegal aliens, to take the AIDS blood test, say annually. If they were AIDS-free, they would be given a health card (similar to a driver's license) with an expiration date. One could be required to have a valid AIDS health card, or it would be illegal for employers to pay the employee or for a principal to allow a student to attend school. There are occupations today which require a health card, so this is nothing new. It is just that its use would be expanded.

While the population in general might have to have their card renewed annually, by taking a new AA blood test, those in critical occupations might be required to take it more frequently, say monthly. A required national AA blood test and an "AIDS Health Card" (AHC) would separate the residents of the U.S. into three groups, perhaps with different colored AHC's:

> STAGE 0: Those who tested negative--without AIDS (green card)
>
> STAGE 1: Those who tested positive but without symptoms (yellow card)
>
> STAGE 2: Those with symptoms (red card)

Those in STAGE 2 would need to be isolated, preferably in private facilities.

ISOLATING OF AIDS VICTIMS

The consideration of isolating AIDS victims, to varying degrees, is a very difficult subject.   In fact, in a recent press conference, when asked if he would send a child of his to a school with an AIDS victim, President Reagan had this to say:

I'm glad I'm not faced with that problem today.   I can well understand the plight of the parents, and how they feel about it.   I also have compassion, and I think we all do, for the child that has this, and doesn't know, and can't have it explained to him why somehow he is now an outcast and can no longer associate with his playmates and schoolmates.

On the other hand, I can understand the problem of the parents. It is true that some medical sources have said that this cannot be communicated in any way other than the ones we already know and which would not involve the child being in the school.   And yet medicine has not come forth unequivocally and said we know for a fact that it is safe.   And until they do, I think we just have to do the best we can with this problem.   I can understand both sides of it.

I am sure that the President has had detailed briefings on AIDS and is privileged to information about this disease not available to the public. He would also like for the public not to panic over AIDS. Here was his golden opportunity. He could have said that he **would** send a child of his to school with children who had AIDS, with no reservations. Why did he not say that? Because he is a man of truth, and the facts that he knew prevented him from saying this. He knew it was not safe.

In spite of this, there are some communities, such as Los Angeles, who have passed laws saying that it is illegal to discriminate against someone with AIDS in housing, employment, attending school or in any other way. Thus, the children with AIDS in those communities have a legal right to freely attend school with noninfected children.

There are other communities passing laws that go in the opposite direction, where the child with AIDS is taught separately, in isolation, but is still given an education.

In New York City, in the fall of 1985, the school board declared that there was an unnamed student with AIDS attending an unnamed school. This set off protest among the parents who did not want their children exposed in that way. These types of protests will continue, in my opinion, until the surgeon general, the Centers for Disease Control and other prestigious medical authorities unanimously declare that AIDS cannot be caught by the exchange of body fluids, such as saliva.

Children, and even those in high school, can be rowdy and scuffle and fight. Occasionally, one child will bite another and even draw blood. What if the child doing the biting has AIDS? His saliva, which contains the AIDS virus, could go directly into the bloodstream of the other child. Of course, there are numerous ways for students to exchange blood. For example, if one has a nosebleed and comes into contact with another who has an open scratch. Sports, such as football, can generate scraped areas that are open to infection by AIDS viruses from another player.

Our hearts really go out to young people with AIDS. They need an opportunity to learn and to lead a happy and productive life as long as they can, before they die of AIDS, but one must weigh those needs against the rights of the vast majority of the people without AIDS, who do not want to contract it. It will eventually boil down to a choice between an individual's rights or the rights of the majority.

POSSIBLE SCHOOL ALTERNATIVES

If the AIDS epidemic continues, and 20 to 25 percent of the students wind up with AIDS, then some alternatives to regular classroom school will have to be considered. One of these alternatives would be to have the teachers teach in front of a video camera, with each grade level being broadcast on a separate UHF frequency, or cable channel; the students would receive these broadcasts and do their classwork in the privacy of their own homes. An alternative to this approach would be the use of video tapes on home video players.

This would be very unfortunate, since part of the value of an education is the social contact with one's peers and the interaction between student and teacher. However, AIDS may force us to move to a more isolated type of education technology.

WHAT ABOUT CIVIL RIGHTS?

Many will question a national AA blood test or quarantine because of civil rights. In order to address that question, we need to step back in time. At one time, each man lived in his own cave and did his own thing. However, as people began to live in communities, of necessity, they had to give up some of their individual rights.

For example, if a large boulder rolled down and blocked the only path into the village, and it was far too big for any one man to move, all of the men in the village would have to get together and collectively move it. One man may have wanted to do something else at the time of the "boulder moving." But the price of being part of that community meant giving up one's individual rights in this area.

Similarly, to be a citizen of the U.S., you have to give up your right to do anything at anytime. You have to agree not to murder, not to crash your car into someone else's and to obey the laws of the land. If someone is not willing to give up his individual rights (to murder, etc.) for the common good, then he does not belong in that society, and we take him out by force and confine him.

If the taking of an AA blood test by everyone or the isolation of infectious individuals is necessary for the common good, which is, in this case, controlling the spread of AIDS, then all citizens and residents of the U.S. must comply or they do not belong in this society.

Never before, in plagues of flu, polio and tuberculosis, has anyone had the gall to say, "I refuse to be quarantined--to h--- with the common good and the health and lives of others." That would have been unthinkable. I believe it is equally unthinkable with regard to AIDS. AIDS is a medical health issue and must be treated as such. AIDS is **not a civil rights** issue. We must do what is best for the health of the majority of the citizens of this country.

IF WE WERE TO QUARANTINE

The danger to the average citizen will have to increase substantially before public demand for action and isolation will be heard. How soon that demand will come and what actions will be taken is impossible to forecast. However, the sooner the actions are taken and the stronger the actions, the better the chance to control AIDS.

If one of the actions decided upon is to quarantine or isolate those with AIDS, those in STAGE 2 would need to be isolated, preferably in private facilities. This could be done by converting some hospitals or hospital wings into "AIDS only" areas. Perhaps religious groups will be able to provide for them, as they have in past plagues. An alternative would be housing in government-provided facilities, such as old Army bases. Research labs looking for a cure for AIDS could be housed in the same buildings, so that they would be near the patients for testing.

It is those in STAGE 1 who present the major dilemma, since there may be millions of them. Perhaps it should be left up to the local community to decide whether or not to allow them to attend school and continue working. The individual state should determine if a green card is required for a marriage license.

If someone in STAGE 1 is fired because he or she has a yellow card, then he should be eligible for the same government benefits as those with AIDS--STAGE 2.

None of these issues are pleasant to deal with and there are no perfect answers that will please everyone. However, if the AIDS epidemic is to be controlled at all, isolation must be a part of the solution.

7

THE EFFECT OF AIDS ON MORALITY AND SOCIETY

The history-changing plague of AIDS will most likely permeate every facet of our society before it is all over. It has already totally changed the society of Hollywood.

In Hollywood, rather than giving everyone kisses on the lips, as was done in the past, everyone is "air kissing." AIDS is the number one topic of converstion there. Cher has lost three friends already to AIDS. Almost everyone in Hollywood, including Shirley Maclaine and Phyllis Diller, has at least one friend who has the disease. Tony Perkins says that he keeps the telephone numbers of his friends with AIDS on his bulletin board so that he does not forget to call them.

Many of the actresses now say that they do not want to kiss anyone, whether he be straight or gay. They take this attitude because they do not know who the man has been with in an intimate way in the recent past. The screen actors guild has supported this, based on the clause in their contract about hazardous conditions. This will also change the type of movies and television shows being produced. There will be far fewer kissing and passionate scenes.

Actress Sharon Gabet who appeared on the ABC program "The Edge of Night," learned that one of her "on-camera lovers" had died of AIDS, after having left the show. All of this has made the whole of Hollywood very skittish, even about intimate kissing scenes.

THE SEXUAL REVOLUTION WILL END

As we look at the sexual revolution, we need to think about revolutions in general. A revolution is a massive attempt to overthrow the status quo. Sometimes revolutions succeed, and sometimes they fail. It looks like the sexual revolution in America is doomed to ultimate failure. Ten years from now, the free-swinging life-style of the 60's, 70's, and the first half of the 80's will be over and, sexually speaking, America will be living in a very puritanical way.

The "swinging singles," who previously have done a great deal of bed-hopping or "sleeping around," will soon bring that type of activity to an end, as they come to realize that they potentially can acquire AIDS from any new sexual partner. This is even worse than if one knew that one might acquire cancer from any new sexual partner, because many types of cancer can be cured, but there is no cure for AIDS. A night of pleasure could lead to ultimate death, within a very few years. The price is too high, and even the swinging singles will not be willing to pay that price. They will become the "celibate singles." Getting a divorce in order to participate in the free sexual lifestyle of singles will lose its appeal.

The vast majority of abortions are by single women. There are only a handful of abortions by married women or as a result of rape. As the singles (and let us include junior high and high school students here) begin to avoid sex because they can acquire AIDS through it, the number of pregnancies of single women will decline dramatically. As these decline, so will the number of abortions.

Within ten years, it would not surprise me to see the present millions of abortions each year decline to just a few. Regardless of what the pro-life groups do or do not do, the abortion issue is going to go away on its own, because of the history-changing nature of AIDS. Single people simply will not be having sex and, therefore, there will not be large numbers of single women getting pregnant.

MARRIED COUPLES WILL
BECOME FAITHFUL

In recent years, there has been a great deal of extramarital sexual activity. This ranges from the affairs that married people might have to orgies and wife swapping parties. As the married people in America begin to realize that any new sexual partner could potentially give them AIDS, they will stop this type of activity. They will stop these activities not only because they do not want to bring a disease back to their spouse, whom they love, but also because they do not want to die of this dreaded disease.

A CHANGE IN SOCIALIZING AND DATING

There will be a change in dating habits among single people, with the advent of AIDS. Sex between singles will be out and possibly even intimate kissing. It looks as if we are being forced to roll the clock back to the times when holding hands was a very intimate thing, and one kissed for the first time at the wedding ceremony. (Hence, the phrase in most wedding ceremonies, "You may now kiss the bride.")

As this AIDS epidemic progresses, it will become more and more popular to marry a virgin, as we said in Chapter 4. It will be an asset to be guarded and cherished.

In prior centuries, there were no cures for venereal diseases. If one were to get gonorrhea or syphilis, one had it for the rest of his life, went insane from it or died from it. Thus, it was essential to marry someone who was disease-free. In those days, the only way to really ensure this was to marry a virgin.

Today, the best assurance that you are marrying someone who does not have AIDS is to marry a virgin. This is better than the AA blood test, because a person could have AIDS without it having progressed to his or her bloodstream; in this case, the AA blood test would not detect it.

In some cases, AIDS goes directly to the brain. The October 16, 1985 issue of USA TODAY reported Dr. Anthony Fauci, Director of the National Institute of Allergy and Infectious Diseases in Bethesda, Maryland, as saying this, in regard to AIDS:[1]

> "It doesn't surprise me. We've been saying all along that it can infect the brain. Sooner or later we were bound to see a case like this."

The same publication also reported that Dr. Alexandria Beckett, of Boston's Massachusetts General Hospital, commented on an AIDS-caused brain disorder case at an American Psychiatric Association meeting in Montreal:

> She said the man, who is in his late 30s, has lost some brain function, has memory loss and dementia. He is paralyzed on his right side and suffers from depression and paranoia.
> Such symptoms are also found in about 30 percent of AIDS victims. Depression is usually an initial symptom of the disease, but doctors have attributed it to the lethargy and fatigue caused by immune suppression.
> The AIDS virus, HTLV-III, was found in the man's spinal fluid. But no

evidence of the virus was found in the man's bloodstream, and he doesn't have any AIDS symptoms, Beckett said.

Also, in prior centuries, if an individual committed adultery (had sexual relations with anyone other than his or her marriage partner) divorce almost always followed. The reason was that the straying partner could have picked up a venereal disease which was, at that time, incurable. Thus, they could never again have sex, unless the faithful partner was willing to take the risk.

AIDS will change the socializing habits of Americans in many other ways. One is that people will be much more cautious as to whom they have over to join them in a hot tub or a Jacuzzi. It could affect attendance at public swimming pools. At present, it does not appear that AIDS can be spread in pools and hot tubs. However, this could change with further research or if the AIDS virus mutates.

It will change people's attitudes about going out to restaurants to eat. People may become more wary of salad bars and finger foods at potlucks and other social events, where someone with AIDS ahead of them in line could have handled the food before them. More restaurants may require use of clean plates for second trips to buffet lines. There will be much more caution exercised in all of these areas.

CHANGES IN FAMILY CONTACT

There will be many changes within the family. The habit some parents have of finishing the glass of milk that a child left half full or finishing the bit of food left on his plate will likely go by the wayside. This would be especially true if a teenage child might have AIDS because of promiscuous kissing or other sexual activity. It is possible that the dishes and silverware of the teenagers might need to be washed in a way closer to sterilization than those of other family members.

In times past, a parent would rush to assist one of his or her teenage children who had a nosebleed. However, as the AIDS epidemic grows, parents may be more hesitant or certainly more cautious in rendering this type of assistance, without rubber gloves. The same thing would be true if the teenage child cut himself and was bleeding profusely. This is sad, but it could easily happen.

LESS "GOOD-SAMARITAN" ACTIVITIES

One of the unfortunate things that is going to happen because of the AIDS epidemic is that you will see a greatly curtailed number of "good-Samaritan" cases. For example, if someone was drowning and needed mouth-to-mouth resuscitation, at some point in time, as the AIDS epidemic rolls on, the typical good Samaritan will hesitate to give that mouth-to-mouth resuscitation because of fear of acquiring AIDS.

Suppose someone scratched or cut his hand, and thus had an opening in the skin of his hand. If he were to stop to help an accident victim, he could easily get that person's blood on his hands. If the accident victim had AIDS, this could potentially allow the AIDS virus to enter the bloodstream of the good Samaritan through the cut, and he could get AIDS in this manner. Unfortunately, people are going to begin to hesitate to help accident victims, because of a fear of acquiring AIDS. Ambulance personnel and paramedics are already very concerned about this, and many wear rubber surgical gloves and other protective clothing.

Another instance would be if someone were to get something clogged in his windpipe; the good Samaritan who normally would have reached into that individual's mouth to try to dislodge whatever was caught, might hesitate to do so, because of the potential danger that this person may have AIDS (and, thus, AIDS viruses in his saliva). The AIDS viruses could go into cuts in the hands of the good Samaritan or the victim could accidentally bite his rescuer. We could go on with other examples, but you can see how "good Samaritan" activity is likely to decrease, as the number of AIDS victims increases.

CHANGE COMING
TO THE SCHOOL SYSTEMS

As we have seen, the admitting of AIDS-infected children to public schools will become a progressively hotter issue. My forecast is that eventually these students will be excluded from the regular public school system. This means that there will have to be separate schools established for AIDS victims, isolated study cells provided, or video teaching instituted.

As we mentioned earlier in this book, with the video revolution in its infancy, one of the most likely candidates in the long run will be to go to video teaching of children. Again, these video tapes either could be played in the student's home or they could be shown on cable or UHF channels. If the classes were broadcast, this would eliminate the possibility of electives during regular class hours; it would mean that all the students in a certain grade level would be taking the same subjects by the same teachers. Elective courses could possibly be broadcast during the off hours, such as late afternoon or early evening.

THE MORALS OF AMERICA
WILL IMPROVE

As we have seen, sex between single people is going to die out as the AIDS epidemic increases. Those who continue their promiscuous sexual activity will all eventually get AIDS and die, and those who abstain will continue to abstain, for fear of getting AIDS, among other reasons.

Adulterous affairs by married people and sexual partner exchanges will become a thing of the past. Those who continue to do this will ultimately get AIDS and die, and others will return to a higher morality.

AIDS has been termed by many as God's judgment upon homosexuals. If you want to consider it God's judgment, I would rather look at it as God's judgment upon all immoral sex. According to the Scriptures, sex should only occur between married people. It looks as if God is bringing us back to the point of abiding by this, "or else"--and that "or else" is to acquire AIDS.

AIDS has already affected the morals of America. The business of prostitutes has dropped off considerably, since the fact has been publicized that you can get AIDS from one of them, if she is infected (AIDS--STAGE 1). Homosexual bathhouses are being shut down.

The deadly plague of AIDS undoubtedly will have an even more significant impact on society and morality in years to come.

8

AIDS AND RELIGION

First and foremost, churches and other religious organizations need to show love and compassion to those with AIDS. They need to provide leadership in this area.

As we saw in the previous chapter, the AIDS epidemic (plague) will very likely bring America back to the morals of Judeo-Christianity, without the help of ministers or rabbis. Neither in the Old Testament nor in the New Testament was promiscuous sex permitted. In the Old Testament, a man could have multiple wives, but he was never permitted to go around and have "casual" or "recreational" sex with anyone he wanted. He was only permitted to have sex with a woman who was his wife, whom he was committed to care for, for the rest of her life.

It is interesting that the same thing was true of most primitive tribes. Even if they were allowed multiple wives, sex outside of the marriage bed was usually considered taboo. Most primitive tribes would never allow promiscuous sex, just for recreation. It was restricted to marriage partners or, in some cases, to those who were going to be married, but then marriage was a required fulfillment.

Whether based on religion or primitive intuition concerning what is right or wrong, the pattern through the centuries has been to restrict sex to the marriage relationship. Now it appears as though we are being forced, perhaps by God, to obey the regulations set forth in the Old and New Testaments.

However, causing a return to the biblical patterns of sex is not the only way that AIDS is going to affect the religious life of Americans and peoples of other nations.

MANY WILL TURN TO GOD

Frequently, it requires tragic circumstances for individuals to turn to God. Of course, we have all heard the old saying that "there are no atheists in foxholes." When all else fails, and our human resources become inadequate, then at last men turn to the only true source of help, their Creator.

This was the experience of Rock Hudson, who sought God intensely for the last weeks of his life. His interest in religion grew steadily. I spoke with Toni Phillips, one of Hudson's nurses, who said that two of his nurses were born-again Christians. Acording to her, Hudson prayed with her to accept Christ on September 14, 1985, about three weeks before his death. After that time, she said his personality changed and what swearing he did came to an end.

She feels that in order to help AIDS victims come into a right relationship to God, we need to love them and have compassion and not to condemn them.

The evening before Rock Hudson died, he held a small get-together for the four nurses who took turns caring for him. It was to honor one of the nurses who was going to Ethiopia to do relief work.

One of the nurses had a video tape of an evangelistic meeting, wherein Ken and Gloria Copeland prayed for Hudson by his real name. This greatly touched Hudson. After watching the video, the nurses reported that Hudson confessed that his life had not been perfect by any standard, but that he felt at one with his God. Then they all gathered around his bed, and he joined them in a time of prayer. Carolyn Fortson, the other Christian nurse, said that there was a real sense of the presence of God during their prayers.

The next morning, Hudson asked the nurse who was on duty to let him sit up in an easy chair so he could look out the window. After going back to bed, he rested for an hour or so, then he looked up at his nurse, smiled and said, "I feel okay. I am at peace with God."

A short while later he lost consciousness. Without ever coming out of that coma, Rock Hudson died one hour later. Thus, his last words were, "I feel okay. I'm at peace with God."

As the AIDS epidemic grows, we will see more and more people, like Rock Hudson, turning to God. As they turn to God in prayer, they are trusting that their prayers will be heard and answered. To be sure that those prayers are heard, we need to examine what the accepted document about God, the Bible, has to say about God answering prayers.

The Bible records case after case in which people turned to God for help, and He required something of them first. The same thing could be true in the case of AIDS victims, their families, or even people who are concerned about getting AIDS. We need to look at what the Bible says God might require of an individual.

GOD'S PREREQUISITE FOR ANSWERING PRAYERS

We think of God hearing all prayers and that is true, in the sense that God hears all of the conversations of everyone, including Hitler and Stalin, and even the most vile criminal who lives today. But for God to "hear" a prayer in a biblical sense, with an obligation to answer, there are some prerequisites pointed out in the Scriptures themselves. Solomon, who was considered by all to be the wisest man who ever lived, had this to say in one of his proverbs:

29 The Lord is far from the wicked
But He hears the prayer of the
righteous.

--Proverbs 15

The wisest man of all time is telling us here that God hears the prayers of the righteous, but not those of the wicked. This wise man, Soloman, goes on to tell us that the prayers of those who will not listen (hear and obey) to the laws of God are even an abomination to God:

9 He who turns away his ear from
listening to the law,
Even his prayer is an abomination.

--Proverbs 28

David--who is revered by Christians and Jews alike--had similar things to say:

18 The Lord is near to all who call
upon Him,
To all who call upon Him in truth.
19 He will fulfill the desire of those
who fear Him;
He will also hear their cry and will
save them.
20 The Lord keeps all who love Him;
But all the wicked, He will destroy.

--Psalms 145

This passage of Scripture is a heavy one, because it tells us that we must call upon God in truth. We must fear Him and love Him in order for our prayers to be answered. These things are not comfortable to think about, but they are what the Bible actually says. However, the Scriptures also inform us that at any time an individual can turn away from the things that separate him and his prayers from God and can turn to God, Who will gladly receive him.

Jesus Christ, the greatest rabbi (teacher) of all times, makes it even clearer in the book of John, when he says this:

> 31 "We know that God does not hear sinners; but if anyone is God-fearing, and does His will, He hears him. . . ."
>
> --John 9

Here Jesus Christ tells us clearly that God does not "hear" prayers of those who are living independent of Him or who are rebellious toward Him. In today's vernacular, this would be "doing your thing" rather than doing God's thing. But Jesus tells us that God only "hears" those who fear Him and do His will.

Since so many people will be crying out to God as the AIDS epidemic accelerates, these prerequisites are things we need to realize, if we want our prayers to be "heard." It would be in order for us to examine ourselves to see if we meet the prerequisites of being righteous, fearing

God, loving Him and not living independent of Him (not doing our own thing).

There is another thing that should be considered while we are discussing prerequisites to having our prayers answered. Jesus Christ said that we should pray to God in his name--that is, possessing the name of Jesus as believers in him and followers of him:

> 16 "You did not choose Me, but I chose you, and appointed you, that you should go and bear fruit, and that your fruit should remain, that whatever you ask of the Father in My name, He may give to you. . . ."
>
> --John 15

> 23 "And in that day you will ask Me no question. Truly, truly, I say to you, if you shall ask the Father for anything, He will give it to you in My name.
> 24 "Until now you have asked for nothing in My name; ask, and you will receive, that your joy may be made full. . . ."
>
> --John 16

This is an incredible claim from this greatest of Jewish teachers, who claimed to be God's only Son. He claimed that if we met the other prerequisites and asked anything in his name, he would do it. To see if this might be true, we need to look further at the person of Jesus Christ to see who he was, to see if he could be--as he claimed to be--the only key to having our prayers answered.

WHO WAS/IS JESUS CHRIST?

Let me explain what is in my heart, as we look at the historic person of Jesus Christ.   As this AIDS epidemic spreads and intensifies, you and I are going to need an internal peace to see us through and to eliminate fear.

Jesus Christ claimed to have a key role to play in an individual making his peace with God.   According to historians, Jesus Christ is the most influential person in history.   We have two national holidays dedicated to him, our daily newspaper is dated from his birth and thousands of hospitals and orphanages have been built in his name.   Therefore, every thinking individual at least needs to examine, with an adult mind, what he had to say and decide who he was:

6   Jesus said to him, "I am the way, and the truth, and the life; no one comes to the Father, but through Me.
7   "If you had known Me, you would have known My Father also; from now on you know Him, and have seen Him."
--John 14

In beginning to look at Jesus Christ, we must first realize that Christians did not get together and decide that theirs was the only religion. The founder of Christianity, Jesus Christ himself, made the claim we just read.

What would you think of Billy Graham if he stood up and made a claim that he was the only way to God? You would think that he was deluded or had gone crazy. Jesus Christ similarly must have been either deluded or crazy OR He was the Son of God and this claim was actually truth. As we have seen, Jesus also claimed that he could do anthing for anyone. In other words, he claimed that he could answer prayer:

13 "And whatever you ask in My name, that will I do, that the Father may be glorified in the Son.
14 "If you ask Me anything in My name, I will do it. . . ."

--John 14

What would you think if the Pope were to make this claim, that if we ask anything in his name, he will do it? Again you would think that he was either a conman or insane. Similarly, Jesus Christ either had to be insane, a conman, or he was in fact the Son of God and he actually can do whatever we ask in his name.

The Bible verse that is probably the most familiar in the world tells us what Jesus said to Nicodemus, a ruler of the Jews:

16   "For God so loved the world,
that He gave His only begotten Son,
that whoever believes in Him should not
perish, but have eternal life . . . ."
                                        --John 3

What if Norman Vincent Peale made this
claim that whoever believed in him would
have eternal life?   We would think that he
was claiming the impossible and belonged in
an insane asylum.   In the very same way,
Jesus Christ either belonged in an insane
asylum or he actually was God's Son and he
can give everlasting life to those who
believe in him.

We could go on and on examining similar
claims that Jesus Christ made.   Some people
think that Christ was just a good teacher, a
good rabbi, a good prophet or a good man.
That is an impossible alternative.   If the
things we have read that he claimed are lies
(not true), then he was a very evil man, or
crazy.

On the other hand, if these things are
true, then he was the Son of God.   It is a
binary (two-way) choice.   Either he was a
conman, deluded and crazy OR he actually
was the Son of God.   It is impossible for
him to be just a good teacher or a good
prophet.   After reading the claims that
Jesus Christ made, I do not believe that a
thinking man would attempt to place him in
the category of a being a very good person
but not the Son of God.

Let me pause as we reflect on this. If someone told me that he had examined the evidences (had read the New Testament documents with an adult mind) and concluded that Jesus was crazy, I could shake his hand and respect that person intellectually. On the other hand, if someone told me that he had examined the evidence and concluded that Jesus was the Son of God, I could equally respect him. Jesus himself left us no other alternative, for if all of these claims are false (lies), then he was evil and not good.

Whoever Jesus Christ was, what does this have to do with AIDS? We are looking at having peace (through a right relationship to God) during the AIDS plague. I am not trying to proselytize anyone, but I am encouraging everyone to find this peace. I personally tried to find it in many different directions with no positive results.

Finally, as a scientist, I decided to look objectively at Jesus Christ and his claims. I saw that anyone could make such claims, but how would you prove or disprove them? Christ himself gave us the method of validation.

He told his disciples that the way that he was going to prove that he was the Son of God, and that all of the claims that he was making were true, was by coming back to life three days after being killed. That was to be his supreme validation for all of the things he had claimed during his lifetime. It is this resurrection from the dead that we celebrate at Easter. If Christ did not rise from the dead, then Easter is a farce and all Christians are fools.

Thus, we see that Christianity stands or falls on the resurrection. We do not have the space to go into an examination of the claimed resurrection of Jesus Christ here, but I have written a booklet on that subject, entitled "EXAMINING THE EVIDENCES FOR THE RESURRECTION." If you are interested in pursuing that, it is available from:

Omega Ministries
P. O. Box 1788
Medford, OR 97501

In that booklet, I examine the evidence, both pro and con, that Jesus Christ rose from the dead. After looking at the evidence objectively, I was forced to conclude that indeed Christ was raised from the dead and, thus, all of his claims were true. Since he claimed that he was the only means to come to God, I had to accept him as the Son of God. When I did that, I had the peace of God and my prayers began to be answered.

My prayer is that each of you reading this book will have this peace through the AIDS plague and that your prayers will be answered, as you come into a right relationship to your God and Creator.

If you are not sure that you are in the proper kind of relationship with God, and you would like to have a close personal relationship with Him through Jesus Christ, I would encourage you to read Appendix A, entitled "How to Have It." This can help you settle the matter in your heart so that you can **know** that you are rightly related to God, and therefore He can and will hear your prayers and will answer them.

THE AGES IN THE BIBLE

Moving from the personal to the universal, we see that the Bible divides history into "ages." The first giant age ended when God intervened on planet earth and gave the ten commandments. Then the rules changed about how one comes into a right relationship with God. The second giant age ended when God again intervened on planet earth and sent His only begotten Son, Jesus Christ, and then once again the rules changed about how one comes into a right relationship with God the Father.

The Bible tells us how our current age will end, when Christ returns in power and glory. The next age will be a one-thousand-year period of time, during which Christ will rule and reign here on the earth and there will be absolute and perfect peace.

There were 330 specific prophecies in the Bible about how the previous age would end and what the Messiah would be like. These were actually 60 major prophecies and 270 variations on those. Jesus Christ fulfilled 330 out of 330, which is essentially an impossibility, mathematically speaking.

Let's imagine for a moment the likelihood of just five characteristics all occurring. For example, say that someone was going to become president of the United States, his first name was going to be Ralph, he was going to be blonde, he would have played football at Notre Dame and his wife's name would be Ruth. What is the probability of all of those things happening? Very remote, and that is with only five characteristics.

If we had 330 characteristics, the likelihood of all of them occurring has about the same probability as if there were an explosion in a print shop (given adequate type) and all of the type were to fall down into the entire works of Shakespeare, without a single error in words, capitals, or even punctuation. The probability of Christ fulfilling all 330 out of 330 prophecies is the same probability of such a print shop accident occurring.

Since the Bible is so accurate concerning how the previous age would end, we can have a high degree of confidence in its prophecies concerning how this current age will end. We are not talking about the end of the world, but just one age ending and another beginning.

Just as God brought the plagues on Egypt, the Bible says God is going to bring many plagues upon the earth as this age is ending, prior to the return of Jesus Christ in power and glory. We cannot get into the details of all of these plagues here, but they are covered in my book THE COMING CLIMAX OF HISTORY.[1] I would simply refer you to that work for the details of how the Bible says this age will end and history will come to a climax.

There are many plagues coming on the earth, according to the Bible, and these could occur within the lifetime of many who will read this book. For an individual to go through these alone, without Jesus Christ, would be a terrible thing. This is one of the reasons why I encourage people to come into a right relationship with God through His Son, Jesus Christ.

Just as God protected Daniel in the lions' den and Shadrach, Meshach, and Abednego in the fiery furnance, God is going to protect HIS people from much that is coming upon the earth and, if they accidentally acquire AIDS, it is possible that He will even miraculously cure them of that dreaded disease. We discuss this further in Appendix B, "A Further Word to Christians."

THE ROLE OF CHURCHES IN AIDS

Churches could play a significant role in the AIDS plague, if they are willing. As we have mentioned, AIDS patients will need hospitals or someplace to go and die gracefully. Just as churches in past decades have established old folks homes and orphanages, soon there will be a crying need for the establishment of AIDS hostels. In these hostels, the churches could not only minister to the AIDS patients physically, but also spiritually, in a way that secular housing units could not do.

Also, as many turn to God because of the agony of the AIDS plague, they are going to be looking for spiritual counseling and spiritual guidance--things that churches are really designed to provide. We could see crowds at churches, bulging the walls in coming years, with people eager and hungry to turn back to God.

Then, in general, the churches can provide moral leadership as the morals of this country become much more pure, not necessarily by choice, but because of the fear of AIDS. By and large, churches today do not preach celibacy. They turn their head at premarital sex and other sexual sins. One of the reasons for this is that many pastors are not living a sexually pure life. If they are single, many of them are not celibate and if they are married, many of them are not faithful to their spouses. Church leaders need first to clean up and purify their own act and then be able to provide moral leadership to their congregations and parishes. Finally, they can provide moral leadership for the nation.

AIDS is going to be an incredible window of opportunity for the churches, if they simply move forward and use the opportunity. Years ago the churches lost their moral leadership of this nation.

Perhaps this is one final chance to regain it.

9
QUO VADIS?

As a young man, I saw a movie entitled "Quo Vadis?" which means "Where are you going?" We can well ask ourselves that question in connection with AIDS, both individually and as a nation.

Many of the things in this chapter will simply be summarizing what we have covered in the rest of the book, with some additional thoughts. Let us first review what you as an individual can do.

WHAT YOU AS AN INDIVIDUAL CAN DO

One of the first and foremost things that you can do as an individual is to protect yourself from getting AIDS. We devoted the entire fourth chapter to this subject. All authorities may not agree with everything in that chapter. However, many of them do and you as an individual have a choice as to whether to be protective of yourself and your family or less careful in your protection. This is an individual decision that I cannot make for you, but, as for me and my house, we are going to be very protective but not paranoid.

Another thing you can do is to pray that the plague of AIDS will be stopped short and not run its full course. You can pray for our national leaders, that God will give them wisdom as to what laws to enact to combat this plague and will cause them to act quickly and decisively. Pray that a cure might be found for AIDS. Pray that God will comfort those with AIDS and their loved ones.

I would encourage you to write your congressman, your senators, the president, and the surgeon general, and give them your input as to what you want done about AIDS on the national level.

House of Representatives
Washington, D.C. 20515

U. S. Senate
Washington, D.C. 20510

The President
White House
Washington, D.C. 20500

The Surgeon General
Dept. of Health and Human Services
Washington, D.C. 20201

On the state level, you can write your governor, state legislature representatives and state health department. On the local level, you can telephone your local health authorities and city council. You can encourage these leaders to take appropriate action and to take it early enough to do some good.

Since we believe that AIDS will add to the already inflationary pressures in the U.S. economy, you could restructure your financial affairs to prepare for the coming inflation.

Certain services are going to be highly in demand, and thus the prices are likely to skyrocket. Because of this, you may want to consider, for example, paying now for your funeral and burial expenses, so that when the time comes and the prices are exorbitant, even if you die from natural causes, your family will be protected.

In general, you can become appropriately concerned over the epidemic of AIDS and you can get your friends concerned. However, avoid panic and hysteria. What you do should be done in a very thoughtful and rational manner.

WHAT WE, AS A NATION, CAN DO

AIDS, a major health hazard to our nation, has been around for four or five years and the government has done nothing to stop or even slow down its spread. Perhaps they are hoping that science will come up with a "quick and complete" cure. AIDS researcher, Dr. John Seale of London says that from what we know about the nature of the virus and similar viruses, the likelihood of having a vaccine that is effective in the twentieth century is, in his view, virtually zero, and the likelihood of having a cure is even less.

I am sure the Soviets would love to see AIDS spread as fast as possible in the U.S. By our government doing nothing, they are pleasing the Soviets, while endangering our citizens and residents.

If the public demand for governmental action becomes loud enough, our government will finally decide to act. There are a number of things we have discussed that they could do.

The first thing they should do is to stop sugarcoating the AIDS epidemic and tell the citizens the truth. The reason they are not doing this is because they are afraid of panic and hysteria. However, it can be done in ways that will not create panic. Education and information are the best defense against AIDS panic.

We know that in controlling an epidemic or plague, the two things that can be utilized are prevention and quarantine. Prevention is basically up to the individual, at the present time. Avoiding the intake of body fluids which contain the AIDS virus is the best and only prevention known. However, when it comes to quarantine, that is 100 percent a government prerogative.

As we discussed in Chapter 6, concerning quarantine, the place to begin would be with identification. This would require a mandatory national AIDS Antibody (AA) blood test for every resident, whether one be a citizen, a legal alien or an illegal alien. Based on the outcome of that test, an AIDS Health Card could be issued, which would have an expiration date similar to the expiration date of a driver's license.

If the general population were tested annually, in order to spread the blood-test load equally across the year, the expiration date would most likely be one's birthday. For those in more critical occupations, such as child care, food handling, health care, or blood bank employees, the test may need to be required more frequently.

The imposition of a national AA blood test would divide the population into those who did not have AIDS, and those who had AIDS--STAGE 1, as well as those with the symptoms, who are in AIDS--STAGE 2.

Then some type of enforced quarantine or isolation of those with AIDS--STAGE 2 should be considered. If the private sector is unable to handle this, then the government, of necessity, would have to provide housing for this isolation. There are many good-quality, abandoned military bases and nearly empty hospitals that could be utilized for this. Those with AIDS--STAGE 2, who were restrained in these AIDS communities, could still lead productive lives as long as they were able, that is until they were hospitalized and died.

These "AIDS retirement villages" would be a bit like leper colonies, in that those who lived there would not be allowed to leave. Rather than looking at it in a negative way, we can look at it in a positive way: this would allow those with AIDS--STAGE 2 to have a place where they can die with dignity, rather than being shuffled from hospital to hospital and nursing home to nursing home, with no one wanting them.

The real problem, as we discussed earlier, is what to do with those with AIDS--STAGE 1, who can infect others. Only time will tell who is correct: those who believe that only a percentage of these will ever develop into AIDS--STAGE 2 or those who believe that all of these will eventually, given enough time, develop into AIDS--STAGE 2.

Until the ultimate fate of those with AIDS--STAGE 1 is known for sure, national legislation concerning them would be unwise. In the meantime, how to treat those individuals should, of necessity, be handled by the local community. The service that the federal government can perform is to identify them through the AIDS Health Card (AHC). If this is done, then an employer, a school official or even someone on a date should legitimately be able to ask to see that AHC.

This would tend to prevent panic from building among U.S. residents. The greatest fear is the fear of the unknown. If people knew which of their fellow workers, their fellow students or even their social contacts had AIDS--STAGE 1, they could be more careful around those individuals. This would do more than anything else to prevent panic.

One problem is that we Americans--and especially the U.S. government--are eternally optimistic.   Even though we were defeated in Vietnam, the average American feels that there is no war that we cannot win. We have a feeling that there is no problem that our scientists cannot solve. We are comfortable, well fed and, up until now, have been relatively disease-free. Consequently, we assume that this good life will go on unchanged forever.

It would take something of disastrous proportions to really get the U.S. populace concerned. It would take a famine, wherein we were actually going hungry, to get us concerned over the plight of the farmers. Millions could reach the AIDS--STAGE 2 category before the citizens will really get concerned about the epidemic of AIDS.

Unfortunately, the earlier that concern is exhibited and action is taken, the better the chance of controlling the AIDS plague. However, the optimism and politics of America may cause those actions to be delayed for many years into the future.

THERE IS MUCH YET TO BE LEARNED

I am sure that just one day after this book comes off the presses, I will wish that I could rewrite portions of it. The information on AIDS is coming forth so fast that I would have preferred not to have written this book until five years from now, when much more will be known. However, by that time the book would do no good at all.

The information in this book is important enough that it needs to be disseminated now, while there is time for the information in it to be useful to people.

Because AIDS information is coming forth so fast, I would need to write a new book each month to keep up with it. This is not possible, so we have done the next best thing. We have started a monthly newsletter about AIDS, to give you the latest findings, the unpolluted truth, and suggestions for your health and longevity. The cost of this newsletter, for purchasers of this book, is just $19 per year. You can write to:

THE AIDS UPDATE NEWSLETTER
P. O. Box 4689
Medford, OR 97501

As an example of new information, recently the AIDS virus has been found in rats and in blood-sucking insects. If the AIDS virus is ever spread by these rodents and insects, the AIDS plague could do far more damage than even I visualize. However, let's not get concerned about that at this point in time, until we know whether or not AIDS can be transmitted in this way. We will keep you you posted in THE AIDS UPDATE NEWSLETTER.

Also, the Pasteur Institute of Paris has some evidence that AIDS can be transmitted in an airborne manner by aerosol (sneeze or cough). This, too, may or may not be true. We will let you know in THE AIDS UPDATE NEWSLETTER.

We have expressed a number of concerns in this book, but in no way do we want it to be a negative book. Even though history was changed through the Spanish flu plague and the bubonic plague, humanity came out on the other side and has gone on to bigger and better things. I have every confidence that humanity will weather this plague of AIDS and come out on the other side. Some of the progress may come in the fields of science and medicine. They may make more rapid progress than envisaged today. On the other hand, it may be like our fight against cancer or the common cold; it may be a protracted battle.

Plagues come to an end when all of the people who are going to die from them have died. Thus, the plague tends to reach a peak on the death toll and then drop off very rapidly, essentially to zero. This is likely the way the plague of AIDS will go. All of those who acquire AIDS because they have been living sexually promiscuous lives, because they are intravenous drug users, or for any other reason, will die off, leaving behind the people who have avoided it and probably have high moral values. It could be that this is a way that God is using to purify the race, to purify humanity.

This is certainly not the end of the AIDS plague nor the fight against it. It is really just the beginning, for there is much yet to do, much more to learn. As we look to God for help, the victory in the end can be ours.

APPENDIX A
HOW TO HAVE IT

If you are reading this, I am assuming that you are not sure that you have received Jesus Christ as your personal Savior and, thus, have come into a good relationship with Father God. Not only is it possible to know for sure that you have this relationship, but God wants you to know. The following is what 1 John 5:11-13 has to say:

11 And the witness is this, that God has given us eternal life, and this life is in His Son.
12 He who has the Son has the life; he who does not have the Son does not have the life.
13 These things I have written to you who believe in the name of the Son of God, in order that you may know that you have eternal life.

These things are written to us who believe in the name of the Son of God, so that we can know that we have eternal life. It is not a "guess so," or "hope so" or "maybe so" situation. It is so that we can know for certain that we have eternal life. If you do not have this confidence, please read on.

In order to get to the point of knowing
that we have eternal life, we need to first
go back and review some basic principles.
First, it is important to note that all things
that God created (the stars, trees, animals,
and so on) are doing exactly what they were
created to do, except man. Isaiah 43 indicates why God created us:

> 7   Everyone who is called by My
>   name,
>   And whom I have created for My
>   glory,
>   Whom I have formed even whom
>   I have made."

Here it says that humans were created
to glorify God. I am sure that neither you
nor I have glorified God all of our lives in
everything that we have done. This gives
us our first clue as to what "sin" is. We
find more about it in Romans 3:

> 23   for all have sinned and fall short
> of the glory of God . . .

This says that we have all sinned and
that we all fall short of the purpose for
which we were created--that of glorifying
God. I have an even simpler definition of
sin. I believe that sin is "living independent
of God." A young person out of high school
can choose which college to attend. If he
makes this decision apart from God, it is
"sin." This was the basic problem in the

garden of Eden.   Satan tempted Eve to eat the fruit of the tree of "the knowledge of good and evil."   He said that if she would do this, she would know good from evil and would be wise like God.   This would mean that she could make her own decisions and would not have to rely on God's wisdom and guidance.   Since you and I fit in the category of living independent of God and not glorifying Him in everything we do, we need to look at what the results of this sin are.

First let me ask you what "wages" are. After thinking about it, because you probably receive wages from your job, you will probably come up with a definition something like "wages are what you get paid for what you do."   That is a good answer.   Now let's see what the Bible has to say concerning this, in Romans 6:

23 For the wages of sin is death, but the free gift of God is eternal life in Christ Jesus our Lord.

Here we see that the wages of sin is death--spiritual, eternal death.   Death is what we get paid for the sin that we do. Yet this passage also gives us the other side of the coin: that is, that through Jesus Christ we can freely have eternal life, instead of eternal death.   Isn't that wonderful?!

But let's return for a moment to this death penalty that the people without Christ have hanging over their heads, because of

the sin that they live in.   In the Old
Testament, God made a rule: "The soul who
sins will die" (Ezekiel 18:4).   If we were
able to live a perfect, sinless life, we could
make it to heaven on our own.   If we live
anything less than a perfect life, according
to God's rule, we will not make it to
heaven, but instead will be sentenced to
death.   All through the Bible we find no
one living a good enough life to make it to
heaven.

This brings us to the place where Jesus
Christ fits into this whole picture.   His
place was beautifully illustrated to me when
I was considering receiving Christ as my
Savior, by a story about a judge in a small
town.

In this small town, the newspapermen
were against the judge and wanted to get
him out of office.   A case was coming up
before the judge concerning a vagrant--a
drunken bum--who happened to have been a
fraternity brother of the judge when they
were at college.   The newspapermen thought
that this was their chance.   If the judge let
the vagrant off easy, the headlines would
read, "Judge Shows Favoritism to Old
Fraternity Brother."   If the judge gave the
vagrant the maximum penalty, the headlines
would read, "Hardhearted Judge Shows No
Mercy to Old Fraternity Brother."   Either
way they had him.   The judge heard the
case and gave the vagrant the maximum
penalty of thirty days or a $300 fine.

The judge then stood up, took off his robe, laid it down on his chair, walked down in front of the bench and put his arm around the shoulders of his old fraternity brother. He told him that as judge, in order to uphold the law, he had to give him the maximum penalty, because he was guilty. But because he cared about him, he wanted to pay the fine for him. So the judge took out his wallet and handed his old fraternity brother $300.

For God to be "just," He has to uphold the law that says "the soul who sins will die." On the other hand, because He loves us He wants to pay that death penalty for us. I cannot pay the death penalty for you, because I have a death penalty of my own that I have to worry about, since I, too, have sinned. If I were sinless, I could die in your place. I guess God could have sent down millions of sinless beings to die for us. But what God chose to do was to send down one Person, who was equal in value, in God's eyes, to all of the people who will ever live, and yet who would remain sinless. Jesus Christ died physically and spiritually in order to pay the death penalty for you and me. The blood of Christ washes away all of our sins, and with it the death penalty that resulted from our sin.

The judge's old fraternity brother could have taken the $300 and said, "Thank you," or he could have told the judge to keep his money and that he would do it on his own. Similarly, each person can thank God for allowing Christ to die in his place and can receive Christ as his own Savior, or he can tell God to keep His payment and that he will make it on his own. What you do with that question determines where you will spend eternity.

Referring to Christ, John 1:12 says:

12   But as many as received Him, to them He gave the right to become children of God, even to those who believe in His name . . .

John 3:16 says:

16   "For God so loved the world, that He gave His only begotten Son, that whoever believes in Him should not perish but have eternal life. . . ."

Here we see that if we believe in Christ we won't perish, but we will have everlasting life and the right to become children of God. Right now you can tell God that you believe in Christ as the Son of God, that you are sorry for your sins and that you want to turn from them. You can tell Him that you want to accept Christ's payment for your sins, and yield your life to be controlled by Christ and the Holy Spirit. (You must accept Christ as your Savior **and your MASTER.**)

If you pray such a prayer, Christ will come and dwell within your heart and you will know for sure that you have eternal life.

If you have any questions about what you have just read, I would encourage you to go to someone that you know, who really knows Jesus Christ as his Savior, and ask him for help and guidance.   After you receive Christ, I would encourage you to become a part of a group of believers in Christ who study the Scriptures together, worship God together and have a real love relationship with each other.   This group (body of believers) can help nurture you and build you up in your new faith in Jesus Christ.

If you have received Christ as a result of reading these pages, I would love to hear from you.   My address is at the end of this book.

Welcome to the family of God.

James McKeever

APPENDIX B

A FURTHER WORD TO CHRISTIANS

This appendix is written to Christians, to those who know that they have a good relationship with God, by having Jesus Christ as their Savior and Master. There are some additional things that God wants you to know about AIDS.

First, we must not discount the possibility that AIDS is a plague sent from God. I am not saying that AIDS is a plague sent from God, but it could be. Certainly everyone agrees that the plagues that came upon Egypt, during the time of Moses, were from God. If God could send plagues in those days, He certainly could still send plagues today, if He so chose.

GOD AND PLAGUES

The human attack on the plague of AIDS will continue and increase in intensity, as the AIDS victims (AIDS--STAGE 2) continue to multiply in numbers. The amount of funds allocated by governments and private organizations to AIDS research and to caring for AIDS victims will continue to increase. However, as these human efforts roll along, we must also seriously look at the relationship of God to plagues in general, and the possible relationship between God and AIDS.

Let us first go back to the plagues that God brought upon Egypt as He was freeing the children of Israel from slavery in Egypt. We see that the Lord was the One who brought the signs and wonders (plagues) upon Egypt, as part of His judgment against them:

>   1   Then the Lord said to Moses, "See, I make you as God to Pharaoh, and your brother Aaron shall be your prophet.
>   2   "You shall speak all that I command you, and your brother Aaron shall speak to Pharaoh that he let the sons of Israel go out of his land.
>   3   "But I will harden Pharaoh's heart that I may multiply My signs and My wonders in the land of Egypt.
>   4   "When Pharaoh will not listen to you, then I will lay My hand on Egypt, and bring out My hosts, My people the sons of Israel, from the land of Egypt by great judgments. . . ."
>
> --Exodus 7

We see that the Lord has said that He would bring these judgments, but many people do not realize that God divinely protected His people from the majority of those plagues.   For example, further in the Exodus account, we read this:

20 Now the Lord said to Moses, "Rise early in the morning and present yourself before Pharaoh, as he comes out to the water, and say to him,' Thus says the Lord, "Let My people go, that they may serve Me.

21 "For if you will not let My people go, behold, I will send swarms of insects on you and on your servants and on your people and into your houses; and the houses of the Egyptians shall be full of swarms of insects, and also the ground on which they dwell.

22 "But on that day I will set apart the land of Goshen, where My people are living, so that no swarms of insects will be there, in order that you may know that I, the Lord, am in the midst of the land.

23 "And I will put a division between My people and your people. Tomorrow this sign shall occur."''''

24 Then the Lord did so. And there came great swarms of insects into the house of Pharaoh and the houses of his servants and the land was laid waste because of the swarms of insects in all the land of Egypt.

--Exodus 8

In the passage above, we see that great swarms of insects came throughout the land of Egypt, but in the land of Goshen--where God's people were dwelling--there were no insects.   Goshen was just one area within

Egypt. Think of it as though Egypt was on the left side of the road and on the right side was the land of Goshen. On the left, there were vast swarms of insects and, on the right side of the road, where God's people were dwelling, there were no insects at all. Thus, we see God's divine protection upon His people, but it was His protection against a plague that He Himself had sent.

Similarly, we see God's protection over the livestock of His people, when He brought a plague on the livestock of Egypt:

1 Then the Lord said to Moses, "Go to Pharaoh and speak to him, 'Thus says the Lord, the God of the Hebrews, "Let My people go, that they may serve Me.

2 "For if you refuse to let them go, and continue to hold them,

3 behold, the hand of the Lord will come with a very severe pestilence on your livestock which are in the field, on the horses, on the donkeys, on the camels, on the herds, and on the flocks.

4 "But the Lord will make a distinction between the livestock of Israel and the livestock of Egypt, so that nothing will die of all that belongs to the sons of Israel."'"

5 And the Lord set a definite time, saying, "Tomorrow the Lord will do this thing in the land."

6 So the Lord did this thing on the

morrow, and all the livestock of Egypt
died; but of the livestock of the sons of
Israel, not one died.

7 And Pharaoh sent, and behold,
there was not even one of the livestock
of Israel dead.   But the heart of
Pharaoh was hardened, and he did not
let the people go.

--Exodus 9

Here we see that all of the livestock of
Egypt died, but in Goshen--where God's
people were dwelling--not even one of the
livestock died. Here again we see that God
sent the plague, but God protected His
people from the plague.

DELIVERANCE FROM GOD'S PLAGUES

Needless to say, one could go on to
look at the many plagues that God has sent
upon the world at various times during the
Old Testament period. This has just been a
glimpse. We would now like to examine
something that God said to King Solomon:

12 Then the Lord appeared to
Solomon at night and said to him, "I
have heard your prayer, and have cho-
sen this place for Myself as a house of
sacrifice.
13 "If I shut up the heavens so that
there is no rain, or if I command the
locust to devour the land, or if I send
pestilence among My people,

14   and **My** people who are called by **My** name humble themselves and pray, and seek **My** face and turn from their wicked ways, then I will hear from heaven, will forgive their sin, and will heal their land. . . ."
                                        --2 Chronicles 7

Here God is telling Solomon that, if the children of Israel are disobedient to Him, He may create a famine--by causing the rain to cease or by sending locusts to devour the produce of the land--or He may send a pestilence (plague), even among His people. In such a case, the plague(s) would come from God.

However, in verse 14 of the preceding passage, God tells Solomon and His people what to do in order to have the plague removed.   God tells His people, who are called by His name, to do four things:

1.   Humble themselves
2.   Pray
3.   Seek His face
4.   Turn from their wicked ways

God is not talking to unbelievers here; He is talking to His people.   "His people" today would be those who believe in Jesus Christ and follow Him, Christians.   God tells them (us) that if they will do those four things, then He will hear from heaven, will forgive their sins, and will heal their land.

An entire book could be written about doing those four things, so God could heal the land, but we will try to touch on each of them just briefly here.

THE FOUR PREREQUISITES
TO GOD'S HEALING

We have just seen what God's people must do before God will heal their land of the plagues that He Himself sends. We certainly want to have our land healed from pestilences (plagues), so let us examine these four things that God's people must do. We will examine these in the personal form, so that you and I can apply them to our own lives.

#1. WE MUST HUMBLE OURSELVES: Since Jesus Christ is the example or the model of what His followers should be, we need to look at the humility of Christ:

5 Have this attitude in yourselves which was also in Christ Jesus,
6 who, although He existed in the form of God, did not regard equality with God a thing to be grasped,
7 but emptied Himself, taking the form of a bond-servant, and being made in the likeness of men.
8 And being found in appearance as a man, He humbled Himself by becoming

obedient to the point of death, even death on a cross.

--Philippians 2

Here we see that God's people are commanded to have the same attitude that Jesus had. He was willing to lay aside all of His divine power and become a humble bondslave of God, even willing to be tortured to death on the cross.

There are many other instances in which we see the humility of Christ, such as when He washed the disciples' feet at the last supper. He played the role of a servant and told them to do the same thing in relation to each other:

12   And so when He had washed their feet, and taken His garments, and reclined at the table again, He said to them, "Do you know what I have done to you?

13   You call Me Teacher and Lord; and you are right, for so I am.

14   "If I then, the Lord and the Teacher, washed your feet, you also ought to wash one another's feet.

15   "For I gave you an example that you also should do as I did to you..."

--John 13

Here again we see Christ, as our example, humbling Himself in performing the duties of a servant to the disciples.

Americans, in general--and this includes us Christians--tend to be very proud. We are full of pride about our homes, our automobiles, our clothes, our possessions. We are very proud of the looks of our church buildings and the size of our church memberships. Pride sometimes leads us to build big monuments (Bible schools or colleges) that will be a memorial to us, even after we die. We do not realize that this pride is one of the most despicable sins against God.

In both the Old and New Testaments, we read about God's total opposition to proud individuals, and what God will do to them:

> 6 But He gives a greater grace. Therefore it says, "God is opposed to the proud, but gives grace to the humble."
>
> --James 4

> 11 The proud look of man will be abased,
> And the loftiness of man will be humbled,
> And the Lord alone will be exalted in that day.
> 12 For the Lord of hosts will have a day of reckoning
> Against everyone who is proud and lofty,

And against everyone who is
    lifted up,
That he may be abased.
                          --Isaiah 2

25   The Lord will tear down the
     house of the proud,
     But He will establish the boun-
     dary of the widow.
                        --Proverbs 15

Here we see that God is opposed to the
proud. He will tear their house down, He
will bring them down low . . . in other
words, He will humble them. We read an
interesting thing that Jesus had to say in
Luke:

11   "For everyone who exalts himself
shall be humbled, and he who humbles
himself shall be exalted."
                            --Luke 14

If you read the preceding verse carefully, you will see that, one way or the
other, you and I are going to wind up
humble. We can either voluntarily humble
ourselves or we can let God crush us
humble, if we remain proud. The place to
begin in humbling ourselves is to realize that
we are nothing without Christ, that we can
do nothing without Him, and that every good
gift that we have comes from Him.   We
need to repent and ask God to forgive us
for taking credit for the things that He has

done and the gifts that He has given to us. If we want our land to be healed from plagues (and this includes AIDS), then God's people must truly humble themselves before Almighty God.

#2. WE MUST REALLY PRAY: The second thing you and I are to do is to earnestly pray.   Almost everyone **knows** enough about prayer; the problem is that we don't put into practice what we know.   We need to pray for our nation, our leaders, the disasters coming upon America, and we certainly need to pray about this AIDS plague. However, casual prayer is not enough.   The Bible tells us that we need to pray fervently:

> 16 Confess your trespasses to one another, and pray for one another, that you may be healed.   The effective, fervent prayer of a righteous man avails much.
>
> --James 5

When is the last time you prayed fervently?   Possibly when you were very sick or when a member of your family was very sick.   We pray fervently if we find out that we have cancer, if we are fired from a job, or if some other disaster strikes.   God is calling His people to pray fervently for our nation and to live righteous lives, because it is the fervent prayer of the **righteous** man that brings about miracles.

In Chapter 8, we examined some prerequisites to having God "hear" our prayers. The Bible also sets forth some guidelines or requirements for us to have our prayers answered. The first of these we read in Chapter 8, but we will repeat it here to refresh your memory:

1.   Pray in Jesus' name:

23   "And in that day you will ask Me no question.   Truly, truly, I say to you, if you shall ask the Father for anything, He will give it to you in My name.
24   "Until now you have asked for nothing in My name; ask, and you will receive, that your joy may be made full. . . ."

--John 16

2.   We must pray believing:

24   "Therefore I say to you, all things for which you pray and ask, believe that you have received them, and they shall be granted you. . . ."
--Mark 11

3.   We must pray in His will:

14   And this is the confidence which we have before Him, that, if we ask anything according to His will, He hears us.

15   And as we know that He hears us in whatever we ask, we know that we have the requests which we have asked from Him.

--1 John 5

4.   Pray without any iniquity in our heart:

18 If I regard wickedness in my heart,
The Lord will not hear; . . .

--Psalm 66

5. Pray having forgiven all:

14 "For if you forgive men for their transgressions, your heavenly Father will also forgive you.
15 "But if you do not forgive men, then your Father will not forgive your transgressions. . . ."

--Matthew 6

6. Pray with right motives:

2   You lust and do not have; so you commit murder.   And you are envious and cannot obtain; so you fight and quarrel.   You do not have because you do not ask.
3 You ask and do not receive, because you ask with wrong motives, so that you may spend it on your pleasures.

--James 4

7.   Keep on praying:

7   Keep on asking and it will be given you; keep on seeking and you will find; keep on knocking (reverently) and the door will be opened to you.

8   For every one who keeps on asking receives, and he who keeps on seeking finds, and to him who keeps on knocking it will be opened.

--Matthew 7, AMPLIFIED

1   Also (Jesus) told them a parable, to the effect that they ought always to pray and not to turn coward--faint, lose heart and give up.

--Luke 18, AMPLIFIED

8.   Obey God and please Him:

22   and whatever we ask we receive from Him, because we keep His commandments and do the things that are pleasing in His sight.

--1 John 3

One additional thought on prayer, before we move on to the next prerequisite on healing our land, is this.   We know that Christ spent long periods of time in prayer; perhaps He wants us to do the same:

35   And in the early morning, while it was still dark, He arose and went out

and departed to a lonely place, and was praying there.

--Mark 1

12   And it was at this time that He went off to the mountain to pray, and He spent the whole night in prayer to God.

--Luke 6

40   And He came to the disciples and found them sleeping, and said to Peter, "So, you men could not keep watch with Me for one hour?
41   "Keep watching and praying, that you may not enter into temptation; the spirit is willing, but the flesh is weak."
--Matthew 26

God's people need to set aside time everyday to get alone with Him and to concentrate and pray fervently. Casual prayers while one is washing dishes or driving down the highway have a place, too, but the prayer that is going to heal the land of America is going to be fervent, concentrated prayer, alone with God.

#3.   WE MUST SEEK HIS FACE: The third thing that we Christians must do is to seek God's face.   We first need to realize that God has spoken to many people face to face.   Two of these were Jacob and Moses:

30   So Jacob named the place Peniel, for he said, "I have seen God face to face, yet my life has been preserved."
--Genesis 32

11   Thus the Lord used to speak to Moses face to face, just as a man speaks to his friend.   When Moses returned to the camp, his servant Joshua, the son of Nun, a young man, would not depart from the tent.
--Exodus 33

As we seek His face, we are seeking a personal relationship with God through Jesus Christ, not a relationship with a religion or even with a church.   The prayer of our hearts should be the same as what was on David's heart:

1   Oh give thanks to the Lord, call upon His name;
Make known His deeds among the peoples.
2   Sing to Him, sing praises to Him Speak of all His wonders.
3   Glory in His holy name;
Let the heart of those who seek the Lord be glad
4   Seek the Lord and His strength;
Seek His face continually.
--Psalm 105

8   When thou didst say, "Seek My face," my heart said to

Thee,
"Thy face, O Lord, I shall
seek."

--Psalm 27

I yearn daily to see (with my spiritual eyes) the face of the Lord and to get to know Him better in a personal way.

#4.   WE MUST TURN FROM OUR WICKED WAYS: As well as humbling ourselves, praying, and continually seeking God's face, the last thing that we are to do is to turn from our wicked ways.   We Christians in America today are not turning from our evil ways, because, by and large, we do not acknowledge that we have any evil ways.   We refer to a "tendency" or an "inclination," rather than calling something sin, as God sees it.

If a Christian today is troubled with the sin of gluttony (overeating), he will most likely say, "I tend to eat too much" or "I have an inclination to eat more than I should" or perhaps even laugh it off with some statement like, "I want to be jolly, and fat people are jolly."   However, if we call overeating what God calls it--the sin of gluttony--then we will be more likely to face it, repent of it, and turn from it.   As we repent, turning from that sin, we must behave in a way that shows we have truly repented:

8 "Therefore bring forth fruit in keeping with repentence; . . ."

--Matthew 3

We Christians have been so brainwashed by television, by the morals of the nation, and by the written media that we have calmly accepted things today that we would have blushed at a number of years ago. God is calling us back to a life of holiness, purity and righteousness.   The church must once again provide moral leadership for the nation.

As God's people, we must ask Him to shine His brilliant searchlight into our hearts and to show us the evil ways that are there:

> 23   Search me, O God, and know my heart;
>   Try me and know my anxious thoughts;
> 24   And see if there by any hurtful way in me,
>   And lead me in the everlasting way.
>
> --Psalm 139

Once God shows us things in our lives that are not pleasing to Him, we need to repent of these things and turn away from our wicked ways.   Only if we do this will God be able to heal our land from the plagues that He has brought or will bring upon it.   The things He shows us may include some of the areas listed in this passage:

> 5   Therefore consider the members of your earthly body as dead to immorality,

impurity, passion, evil desire, and greed, which amounts to idolatry.

6 For it is on account of these things that the wrath of God will come

7 and in them you also once walked, when you were living in them.

8 but now you also, put them all aside: anger, wrath, malice, slander, and abusive speech from your mouth.

9 Do not lie to one another, since you laid aside the old self with its evil practices, . . .

--Colossians 3

Here God tells us to put away even things like anger, filthy language and unholy passion. We need to let God cleanse us, by the blood of Jesus, from all that is unholy.

Unless God's people are willing to do the four things that we have examined, from 2 Chronicles 7:14, and to do them earnestly and intently over a period of time, then things like AIDS could continue to ravage our land.

These four things that we have discussed not only apply to the nation but also to the "land" of an individual Christian. For example, during the drought in Africa, there are documented cases of an individual Christian humbling himself, praying earnestly, seeking God's face and turning from all of his wicked ways. It then rained on his farm, while there was no rain on any of the farms around him. His crops flourished, while the crops of the other farmers died.

God can, and I believe will, heal your personal land and your family, if you do these four things.

PROTECTION DEPENDENT
UPON OBEDIENCE

In most of the plagues of Egypt, the children of Israel were protected simply because they were there. However, in the last plague, they only received God's protection if they were obedient. If they obeyed God and sacrificed a lamb and sprinkled the blood over the doorpost, then they were protected from the death angel. If they did not obey God, then they were not protected and their oldest son died, just as the oldest son of the Egyptian families died.

God wanted to protect Noah from the flood, but Noah's protection was dependent on his obedience. If he obeyed God and built an ark, then he got God's protection. On the other hand, if he had had the attitude of: "I don't need to do anything, God will take care of me anyhow," then I do not think that God would have been under any obligation to take care of him and he likely would have died in the flood, along with everyone else.

Today God is calling His people to obey Him by becoming His bondslaves. Let me just briefly explain what I mean by a bondslave, and why this is relevant to our discussion in this book. A slave is very different from a servant.   A servant gets wages and, therefore, has discretionary spending.   A servant has days off and can do anything he wants on those days. Servants can marry who they want to marry and they have legal rights.

A slave, however, has no rights at all, no money of his own, no possesions of his own, no days off (he is a slave 365 days a year, year after year) and he is obligated to do anything the master tells him to do. The definition of a bondslave in the Bible is found in Exodus 21:1-6.   You can turn there if you wish to read what the Bible has to say about a bondslave.

Essentially a bondslave is a "volunteer permanent slave."   Our concept of slavery is of someone being captured and forced into slavery or being born into slavery.   For someone to walk up to a master and volunteer to become his permanent slave is unthinkable to us.   Yet, God asks His people to volunteer to become His permanent bondslaves.

This whole concept of being God's bondslave is discussed in detail in my book YOU CAN OVERCOME. (See the last pages of this book for ways to obtain YOU CAN OVERCOME, if you are interested.)   You should know, however, that at the end of this age, God is going to do something special for those who are His bondslaves:

2   And I saw another angel ascending from the rising of the sun, having the

seal of the living God; and he cried out with a loud voice to the four angels to whom it was granted to harm the earth and the sea,

3   saying, "Do not harm the earth or the sea or the trees, until we have sealed the bond-servants of our God on their foreheads."

--Revelation 7

Here we see that God seals His bondslaves (bond-servants is not a good translation) on their foreheads.   Later we find out why: He seals them for their protection against the plagues coming upon the earth.   We find one example of this protection two chapters later:

3   And out of the smoke came forth locusts upon the earth; and power was given them, as the scorpions of the earth have power.

4   And they were told that they should not hurt the grass of the earth, nor any green thing, nor any tree, but only the men who do not have the seal of God on their foreheads.

5   And they were not permitted to kill anyone, but to torment for five months; and their torment was like the torment of a scorpion when it stings a man.

6   And in those days men will seek death and will not find it; and they will long to die and death flees from them.

--Revelation 9

Here we see that some locusts come forth that do not swarm over trees, bushes, and grasses and denude them, but they swarm over humans and sting them all over like scorpions sting. It will be so painful that men will yearn to die but won't be able to. However, if you look very carefully at verse 4, those with the seal of God on their foreheads are protected against this plague! So once again, we see the biblical pattern repeating itself: God's protection is dependent on each Christian's willingness to be totally obedient, as a bondslave.

DIVINE HEALING

Almost every doctor has had a case wherein someone was given up as hopeless and was told that he was going to die. There have been many such instances wherein Christians prayed for such an individual and he was miraculously healed.

I personally know of one pastor's wife, who the doctors were operating on for some reason, and they unexpectedly found her body filled with cancer, so they sewed her up and predicted she had just a short period of time to live. A whole host of Christians, myself included, began to pray that God would touch her body, would heal her and would rid her of cancer. Two months later the doctors again opened her up and found absolutely no trace of cancer whatsoever.

While Jesus Christ walked the earth, He caused the deaf to hear, He healed the blind so that they could see, and He healed people with twisted limbs and made them whole.   There was even a case of a man totally paralyzed whom Christ healed, so that he was able to walk freely just as other people.

In the coming years, if Christians are living pure, wholesome lives and they accidentally contract AIDS, through no fault of their own, I believe that through the fervent prayers of righteous men and women, God can and will heal them.   Of course, God can sovereignly heal someone, but He usually moves in answer to prayer.

We need to realize that faith has a great deal to do with healing.   This was true even when Jesus Christ was here on the earth:

> 28   Then Jesus answered and said to her, "O woman, your faith is great; be it done for you as you wish."   And her daughter was healed at once.
>
> --Matthew 15

> 52   And Jesus said to him, "Go your way; your faith has made you well." And immediately he regained his sight and began following Him on the road.
>
> --Mark 10

Another thing to realize is that evidently sometimes a particular sin problem was a hindrance to the healing ministry of Christ. The sin problem had to be dealt with first, before the healing could occur:

2 And many were gathered together, so that there was no longer room, even near the door; and He was speaking the word to them.

3 And they came, bringing to Him a paralytic, carried by four men.

4 And being unable to get to Him because of the crowd, they removed the roof above Him; and when they had dug an opening, they let down the pallet on which the paralytic was lying.

5 And Jesus seeing their faith said to the paralytic, "My son, your sins are forgiven."

6 But there were some of the scribes sitting there and reasoning in their hearts,

7 "Why does this man speak that way? He is blaspheming; who can forgive sins but God alone?"

8 And immediately Jesus, aware in His spirit that they were reasoning that way within themselves, said to them, "Why are you reasoning about these things in your hearts?

9 "Which is easier, to say to the paralytic, 'Your sins are forgiven'; or to say, 'Arise, and take up your pallet and walk'?

10 "But in order that you may know that the Son of Man has authority on

earth to forgive sins"--He said to the paralytic--

11   "I say to you, rise, take up your pallet and go home."

12   And he rose and immediately took up the pallet and went out in the sight of all; so that they were all amazed and were glorifying God, saying, "We have never seen anything like this."

--Mark 2

You notice in this passage that the man's sins were forgiven first, and then the healing took place.   In the situation with the sick man at the pool of Bethesda, after Jesus had healed him, He cautioned him not to sin anymore:

2   Now there is in Jerusalem by the sheep gate a pool, which is called in Hebrew Bethesda, having five porticoes.

3   In these lay a multitude of those who were sick, blind, lame, and withered, (waiting for the moving of the waters;

4   for an angel of the Lord went down at certain seasons into the pool, and stirred up the water; whoever then first, after the stirring up of the water, stepped in was made well from whatever disease with which he was afflicted.)

5   And a certain man was there, who had been thirty-eight years in his sickness.

6   When Jesus saw him lying there, and knew that he had already been a long time in that condition, He said to him, "Do you wish to get well?"

7   The sick man answered Him, "Sir, I have no man to put me into the pool when the water is stirred up, but while I am coming, another steps down before me."

8   Jesus said to him, "Arise, take up your pallet, and walk."

9   And immediately the man became well, and took up his pallet and began to walk. . . .

14   Afterward Jesus found him in the temple, and said to him, "Behold, you have become well; do not sin anymore, so that nothing worse may befall you."

--John 5

Notice carefully verse 14, wherein Jesus tells the man that he should not sin anymore, lest something worse happen to him. Evidentally, Christ made a much stronger connection between sin and healing than we do today.

We can see that if a person has faith and there is not a sin problem separating him and God, then God's divine healing power can be released through the effectual fervent prayers of righteous people, and I believe God can even heal those with AIDS.

HAVE NO FEAR

In connection with AIDS, we need have no fear. We need to act wisely and take all the reasonable precautions that we can and then, as believers in Jesus Christ, we can rest in the Lord and trust in Him. The Bible tells us that perfect love casts out fear:

> **18** There is no fear in love; but perfect love casts out fear, because fear involves punishment, and the one who fears is not perfected in love.
>
> --1 John 4

That perfect love is not your perfect love, but God's perfect love. If you really had any concept of how all-powerful God is, how much He loves you and that, if you are a Christian, He will never leave you nor forsake you, then you would never again fear anything.

VICTORY IN THE END

In the end, God and His Son, Jesus Christ, will win. The victory is ours through Christ Jesus! We can rest in true peace and comfort in this victory:

> **14** But thanks be to God, who always leads us in His triumph in Christ, and manifests through us the sweet aroma of the knowledge of Him in

every place.
15 For we are a fragrance of Christ to God among those who are being saved and among those who are perishing;...
--2 Corinthians 2

35 Who shall separate us from the love of Christ?   Shall tribulation, or distress, or persecution, or famine, or nakedness, or peril, or sword?
36 Just as it is written,
"FOR THY SAKE WE ARE BEING
PUT TO DEATH ALL DAY LONG
WE WERE CONSIDERED AS
SHEEP TO BE SLAUGHTERED
37 But in all these things we overwhelmingly conquer through Him who loved us.
--Romans 8

This says that we are not just conquerors, overcomers in Christ, but we overwhelmingly conquer. So take reasonable precautions, humble yourself before God, pray, seek His face, turn from your wicked ways and, as you walk pure, holy and righteous before Him, He will divinely protect you as His bondslave, and you have absolutely nothing to fear.

However, if you are not willing to be God's bondslave and to walk in a pure and holy way before Him, you may prevent Him from coming to your aid.

REFERENCES

Chapter 1

1. INFLUENZA: THE LAST GREAT PLAGUE (Prodist-Neale Watson Academic Publications Inc., 156 Fifth Ave., New York 10010)

2. "HTLV-III/LAV Disease," JAMA (National Cancer Institute, Bldg. 37, Rm. 6A09, Bethesda, MD 20205) 18 Oct. 1985, Vol. 254, No. 15, p. 2095

3. NEWSWEEK (The Newsweek Bldg., Livingston, NJ 07039) 29 Apr. 1985

Chapter 2

1. "Leading Scientists Sound Global Alarm on AIDS," EXECUTIVE INTELLIGENCE REVIEW (Campaigner Publications, P.O. Box 17726, Washington, D.C. 20041), 11 Oct. 1985, p. 25

2. MORBIDITY AND MORTALITY WEEKLY REPORT (MMWR), (Centers for Disease Control, Atlanta, GA) 13 Sept. 1985

3. MMWR, 4 Jul. 1981; 9 & 16 Jul., 24 Sept. 1982; 2 Dec. 1983

4. MMWR, 12 Nov. 1982; 9 Mar. 1984

5. MMWR, 13 Sept. 1985

6. MMWR, 18 Jun 1982; 6 Jan. 1984; 11 Jan., 27 Sept. 1985

7. MMWR, 11 Jun., 24 Sept. 1982; 4 Mar. 1983; 9 Sept., 22 Jun. 1984; 22 Mar., 3 May, 2 Aug. 1985

8. Department of Human Resources, Oregon State Health Division (1400 S.W. 5th Ave., Portland, OR 97201)

9. "AIDS: A Growing Threat," TIME (Time & Life Bldg., Rockefeller Center, New York 10020) 12 Aug. 1985, p. 43

10. MMWR, 30 Aug. 1985

11. LOS ANGELES TIMES, (Times Mirror Co., Times Mirror Sq., Los Angeles, CA 90053) 16 Aug. 1985

12. STAR, (News Group Publications, Inc., 660 White Plains Road, Tarrytown, NY 10591), 24 Sep. 1985, p. 20

13. "The New Victims," LIFE (Time, Inc., Time & Life Bldg., 1 Rockefeller Center, New York, NY 10020) July, 1985, p. 15

Chapter 3

1. THE MCALVANY INTELLIGENCE ADVISOR (P.O. Box 39810, Phoenix, AZ 85069)

2. R.E. McMaster, THE REAPER (P.O. Box 81369, Corpus Christi, TX 78412)

3. STAR, 24 Sept 1985, p. 21

4. EIR, 11 Oct. 1985, p. 24

5. AIDS IS MORE DEADLY THAN NUCLEAR WAR (NDPC, P.O. Box 17729, Washington, D.C. 20041), Oct. 1985, pp. 2-4

Chapter 4

1. "AIDS Epidemic Explodes," EIR, 18 Oct 1985, p. 53

2. "AIDS: What Women Must Know Now," GOOD HOUSEKEEPING, (Hearst Corp., 959 Eighth Ave., New York, NY 10021) Nov. 1985, p. 246

3. "School and Day Care Policies Pertaining to AIDS," Department of Human Resources, Health Division, 16 Sept. 1985, p. 2

4 "Inpatient Infection Precautions for AIDS Patients," Rogue Valley Medical Center (691 Murphy Rd., Medford, OR) 1985, pp. 1-2

5 MMWR, 30 Aug. 1985, pp. 109-110

Chapter 5

1. WALL STREET JOURNAL (Dow Jones & Company, Inc., P. O. Box 4189, Federal Way, WA 98063), 23 Sept 1985, p. 1

Chapter 6

1. EIR, 11 Oct. 1985, p. 28

Chapter 7

1. USA TODAY, 16 Oct. 1985, p. 10

Chapter 8

1. COMING CLIMAX OF HISTORY (Omega Publications, P.O. Box 4130, Medford, OR 97501, 1982)

THE AIDS UPDATE NEWSLETTER

EDITOR: Dr. James McKeever, Ph. D.

EXECUTIVE EDITOR: René Baxter

- CONTINUOUS UPDATES on the latest developments concerning the vital subject of AIDS

- PLUS current RECOMMENDATIONS on how to protect yourself and those you love

- Unbiased reporting of information from sources around the world

- A MONTHLY publication

- This $39 newsletter is just $19 a year for purchasers of this book

- Use the convenient order form on the next page to subscribe now!

THE AIDS UPDATE NEWSLETTER
P. O. Box 4689
Medford, OR 97501

TO THE AUTHOR

The various services and materials available from James McKeever are shown in summary form on the reverse side. Please indicate your area of interest, remove this page, and mail it to him.

James McKeever would appreciate hearing any personal thoughts from you.

Comments:

ORDER FORM

Dear Dr. McKeever,

Please send me the following:

_____ THE AIDS UPDATE NEWSLETTER
$19 is enclosed for 1-year subscription

_____ copies of this book at $5.95 each for softback or $16.95 for hardback (check should be payable to AIDS UPDATE NEWSLETTER)

TOTAL AMOUNT ENCLOSED $_____

Please send me information about:

☐ Other books you have written

☐ Your speaking at our group or conference

☐ Please read the comments on the other side

Name _____

Address _____

City, State _____ Zip _____

Mail to:

THE AIDS UPDATE NEWSLETTER
P. O. Box 4689
Medford, OR 97501